Juice Dieting In A Healthy Way

A Guidebook To Help You Lose Weight, Get Energy Boost And Perform Body Detox Safely Plus 101 Juice Diet Recipes

Sarah Sparrow

PUBLISHED BY:
Sarah Sparrow
Copyright © 2012

http://JuiceDietTips.com

Table of contents

History of Juicing

Juicing for health or well-being has been performed throughout the dawn of man.   From the earliest records of a human civilization, juicing has been practiced.

One of the earliest juicing recipes came from the Polynesians. They would take the juice from passion fruit and mix it with water. The result was a brisk, refreshing drink that gave the person a burst of energy.   This was immensely popular among the ancient Polynesian island peoples.

It is written in Genesis of the Bible that God makes references to "herb bearing seeds" which prove that biblical-era civilization enjoyed the benefits of juicing.   Furthermore, within the writings of the Dead Sea Scrolls (which were discovered in the middle of the 20th Century) show proven healing methods from juicing. These writings were written by the ancient Jews and Essenes.   Those two civilizations were well-known throughout time as having the most prolific vegetarian diets.

Ancient India had several writings that touted the benefits of juicing.   The medical practice name Ayurveda was first founded in India.   The Ayurveda medicine men would press the juice from fresh fruit, vegetables, and plants.   They would mix these juices with milk, spices and honey to produce not only a highly beneficial and healing medicine, but one that had superb taste.   This form of medicine had several different juicing recipes.   Different recipes would restore the blood, combat fatigue, energy, vitality, the treatment of head lice, stomachaches, gas problems, prevention of gallstones, kidney cleansing, and many more.   Whatever your ailment, the Ayurveda doctor, would have a juicing cure for you.

In 1936, Dr. Norman W. Walker wrote a book title "Raw Vegetable Juices" which preached the benefits of juicing for our modern world.   With the advent of commercial growing for the masses, much of the natural vitamins and minerals found in fruits, vegetables, and plants are lost due to chemicals. Animal meat that was once pure and fed on the plants of the lands, are now tainted with steroids for growth and the pesticides from the plants and grains they consume. The variety of edible fruits, vegetables, and plants is also limited. Commercial farmers of today only grow those plants, fruits, and vegetables that are most cost effective and will produce the most crops. In the modern era, it is estimated that the typical person may only eat a variety of around 20 different kinds of food throughout their life. This is drastically different than during the time of our ancestors.

Our soil itself has even changed. The constant growing on the lands has diminished the minerals and nutrients from the soil. The fertilizers we use to replenish the soil for additional growth are full of chemicals that are not beneficial to our bodies.

Dr. Linus Pauling, owner of two Nobel Peace prizes, have spoken of research that showed the harmful effects of not having the right amount of vitamins and minerals in the human body. He said that many of the ailments, illness and diseases are attributed to this lack within our bodies.

Even our oceans are no resource to regain these natural vitamins and minerals. Over the decades, commercial fishing has depleted the sea life that was once abundant. Boats, both private and commercial, have contributed to pollution in the water which kills or contaminates the sea life that is left.

Indeed, juicing with fresh juices is our only bastion left to feed our bodies the needed nutrients it needs. Juicing will get you back to what our bodies were designed to be—strong and healthy.

Juicing Overview

Regardless of why you want to start juicing, congratulations. You're taking the first steps toward getting a better "you." It doesn't matter the reason. The only thing that matters is that you understand the potential benefits you may gain by incorporating a fresh juicing diet to your eating habits.

There are several items to consider when you decide to partake in a juicing diet or fast. One of the first steps to understand is what you want to accomplish with your juicing efforts. Do you want to achieve a specific result like losing weight? If so, then you need to stick with the fat-loss juicing fasts. Other considerations are if you want to gain energy, fight a specific ailment such as diabetes, look younger, feel younger, or do a total body flush. See? It's not just as uninvolved as grabbing any old fruit, vegetable or plant and getting the juices out of it. The peoples of the ancient world actually had a tremendous thought process in their juicing efforts. What's even more tremendous is that they had to learn all of these "secrets of juicing" by basic trial and error. There were no books to buy off the shelf or expensive laboratories to conduct extensive research on a particular fruit or vegetable.

When particular things were found out by trial and error approach, those were handed down through the generations like sacred family treasures. Each generation gained more knowledge from the previous generation. It took many generations to discover what you'll be able to find out within these pages. Quite a miraculous task if you think about it. Now, back to juicing.

In today's world, grabbing a quick breakfast, lunch or dinner has become the norm. While those quick foods are convenient, they are robbing your body of valuable nutrients on a daily basis. Fast foods are loaded with fat and extremely skimpy on the nutrition scale. It's not entirely your fault. Society and our lifestyles have made it okay for us to eat that way. Fast food chains and convenient stores wouldn't be growing in popularity if society didn't want them there.

Many fast or convenient foods are made with refined white flour. Flour loses over 90 percent of its vitamins and minerals during this refinement process. Those nutrients are desperately needed for your body to build or repair. Many "whole wheat" breads are better, but still lack what is in raw, unrefined wheat flour.

Even much of the meat that we consume in fast or convenient form is not whole, natural meat. Many of them have fillers in them that do nothing more than make 1 pound of meat into 2 or sometimes even 3 pounds of meat, no nutritional value is found in fillers.

In a nutshell, almost everything we eat outside of our homes have been processed, cooked, filled, mashed, or baked until nearly all nutritional value is lost. This doesn't make a reliable source of fuel for our demanding bodies. We need to replace that lost source. Juicing will replace those lost nutrients we need back into our bodies.

That doesn't mean you need to stop enjoying your favorite burger and fries for lunch. What it does mean is that you need to supplement what is lacking by something more than taking a vitamin a day. Juicing will fill this void in your body if done on a regular basis.

By combining several different juices together in a single drink, you will be blasting your body with the ever-needed nutrients it craves. The result will be a more efficiently working system, and you'll reap the benefits from your efforts. Let's take a look at the differences between the three basic styles of juicing.

Juice Diet

A typical juice diet will vary in degrees of strictness. Most juicing diet plans will allow you to eat your normal foods, but also drink unique blends of various fruit and vegetable juice to enhance digestion or burn fat from the foods that you are consuming. Exercise may also be incorporated with these types of juicing diets.

A normal juice diet that also incorporates a healthy well-balanced meal plan will be allowed for almost any person. If you have a specific condition such as diabetes, epilepsy, high blood pressure, or other life threatening condition, you must first see your doctor for individual instructions and help in finding an alternative juicing diet. There are distinct juicing diets that are specifically designed with your condition in mind. Do not try a "normal" juicing diet if you suffer from a severe condition as it may be seriously hazardous to your well-being.

Juice Fasting

The main ingredient in a juice fasting plan is no solid food intake at all. They can range from a 1 day plan up to a 21 day cycle plan. Juice fasting will give positive results in a short amount of time. It also will benefit your body due to the natural cleansing your body will receive from an all liquid diet.

The reason for the cleansing comes naturally. There will be zero amounts of solid food in your digestive tract to process. Therefore, without any digestion of solid foods to do, your body will naturally remove any excess build-up within your digestive walls.

These fasting plans have to be performed with strict self-control. Over the course of the plan or cycle, your body will undergo a drastic change. Headaches, nausea and fatigue, are the key issues to overcome. These types of strict plans are better performed when you're not requiring as much energy from your body in your daily course of events. Most practitioners of this method perform these fasts during a holiday or vacation, so their bodies can rest during that time.

Another item to consider is when you stop doing the juice fast. It's not quite as straightforward as just stopping and eating solid food again. Your body will reject the solid food because it's been accustomed to a pure liquid diet and will treat it like a foreign object. You'll become massively nauseated, sick to your stomach, tired and have headaches. You must slowly introduce solid foods back into your system. This topic will be covered later in this book under "Safe and Healthy Methods of Juicing."

Juice Cleansing

While juicing in general will cleanse your body of toxins and pollutants, there are distinct juice cleansing diets available that will target specific body parts you desire to be cleaned. Not many people realize the benefits of juice cleansing from time to time without actually performing a full juice diet or fast. This kind of juicing is a potent "maintenance plan" for the in-between times you may want to diet or fast.

At times, particular body areas become toxic and may need to be cleansed. This type of juicing targets those areas and removes unwanted pollutants. Human organs are not the only parts that can be specifically targeted for cleansing. Skin, hair, fingernails and toenails along with other areas can be cleansed of unwanted toxins.

Summary

As you can see, there are a few different styles of juicing. Basically saying, there's a juicing plan for every person. You just have to know what you want and check with your doctor for any unknown health concerns. Juicing has been known to make an otherwise unnoticeable condition surface itself during the plan. Juicing removes toxins and, therefore, anything that was masking your condition will surface. Either way, your body will be better once you get your juicing plan underway.

Does It Work and What to Expect

If anyone ever wonders if juicing actually works need only to look toward the life of Jack LaLanne. Although he was a bodybuilder and fitness instructor, he thoroughly believed in the benefits that juicing could provide. He was the father of the Jack Lalanne Juicer that sold millions throughout the globe and was only taken down by pneumonia at the old age of 96. Some of the feats that he accomplished at an elderly age would make other people shudder just training for such a task. However, through fitness and juicing, he managed to accomplish all of which he set out to do.

Besides having Jack LaLanne's personal experience to look toward, you can also dive into the history books about juicing. Ancient civilizations that practiced juicing, which many of them did report a large elderly population. By having an elderly population, which many civilizations did not at the time, shows that juicing keeps humans healthy and provides the longevity that we were designed to have.

Supermodels, actresses and actors, swear by juice fasting, dieting and cleansing. It helps them maintain their weight and keeps their skin complexion looking natural and problem free. It also keeps their hair full and soft, their nails stay strong, and their eyes stay clear and full-colored. Everything that is required of a person that has to "look their best at all times" is provided through a solid juicing regimen.

Athletes from the weekend warrior to the professional utilize the benefits of juicing to enhance their performance. Juicing gives them energy and needed strength to have an edge over their competition. It also has a more inward effect by enhancing their eyesight and hearing. Juicing also allows them to recover from injuries at a much quicker rate. Juicing is one of the only methods allowed by sporting associations that will provide these benefits and enhancements.

There are several studies back by nutrition doctors that have clear evidence that juicing does work. Patients that have been diagnosed with cancer have been shown to have stopped the growth of cancer, reduce the size of cancer or, in the rare case studies, even have the cancer go into remission while on a juicing diet plan. Patients that have been diagnosed with Hepatitis C have been shown to lead a long and disease free life while juicing. The juicing plan provides them the needed nutrients that the disease or condition may be depleting them of, which in turn makes them sick or eventually dies from. When specific plans are designed around the patient's particular area of concern and when done along with a doctor's supervision, miraculous advancements are being recorded.

Signs of juicing working are all around you. People that you may never know to juice may actually be juicing. Anybody that you just assume to be blessed with excellent health probably has some form of juicing going on in their diet. Whether it's something on the mere basic level, such as having a glass or two of orange or apple juice, to performing a juice fast they never discuss. It could be too they consume raw fruits and vegetables on a regular basis and shy away from the fast or convenient food choices. Either way, there is proof in the pudding that juicing does work.

The "Why" Behind Juicing

Studies have shown that juicing fruits and vegetables is the most efficient way for your body to absorb the much needed vitamins, minerals, enzymes and fiber it needs to run in peak performance. With today's hectic lifestyles, it is a highly convenient method to receive the recommended daily intake of the 3 servings of vegetables we need. Mix in some fruit into your juicing diet and you'll also get the recommended daily intake of 5 servings of fruit. Besides its being quick and convenient to get all of the necessary servings, you can mix the juices into your own personal favorite flavors. The sky's the limit for taste and the different blends available can be specifically designed for anybody's palate.

Juicing fruits and vegetables also keep all of the minerals, vitamins, enzyme and fiber intact. Cooking these fruits and vegetables significantly reduces, or all together eliminates, all of these many needed nutrients. By simply juicing them, everything remains intact and ready for immediate absorption into your body and bloodstream.

Enzymes are the single-most essential ingredient for your body to produce energy on the cellular level. Without these crucial enzymes working hard for us, our energy levels are substantially reduced. Without our energy levels high, we become lethargic, irritable and unmotivated. All we would want to do is sleep in order to conserve our energy.

The raw vitamins and minerals that juicing gives help support and build a variety of organs. When mixed right, your juicing blend, can give your entire body the needed protection and building structure to repair many common ailments. From weak hair to poor skin, juicing with the proper blends of fruits and vegetables will rebuild what daily living takes away from us.

The natural fiber that we receive while juicing maintains our digestive system and keeps our bodies processing the food we do intake on a peak performance level. Anything from a sour stomach to constipation can be prevented or cured with a regimen of properly selected fruits and vegetables.

The American Cancer Society has fully endorsed juicing as a method to ward off any potential health problems. Research has proven that, with all the right servings of fruits and vegetables, our bodies build a natural resistance to most ailments, including cancer. All of us our born with cancerous cells within our bodies. What prevents some of us from having full-blown cancer depends not only on our genetic make-up, but on the foods we eat. Partaking in a healthy diet with plenty of fruits and vegetables has shown to aid in battling the cancerous cells.

Our society has developed a frightfully unhealthy diet that consists of foods that are high in fat and cholesterol and not getting enough exercise. By limiting your intake of high fat, high cholesterol foods, while also getting regular exercise of at least 15-30 minutes per day, our bodies will not only be healthier than we ever thought it could feel, it will give us the energy to navigate our way through our daily lives. Let's face it. Our lives are extremely busy in the modern world, and our diets suffer from the lack of healthy eating habits. Mostly due to the lack of time we have for meal planning and eating. We all look for the "quick dinner", "quick breakfast" or the "quick lunch." Even our snack times have become "quick" in nature, and instead of grabbing some fruits or vegetables to nibble on between meals, we're looking for the bag of potato chips from the vending machine. If you set a little time aside in your schedule to juice a satisfying drink and take it with you, then those potato chips won't look quite so appealing to you. A juice drink made from your favorite fruits and vegetables will fill the void that your stomach has in-between meals.

What Results You Can Expect

The first initial result or feeling you will experience is the "flame out" feeling. This feeling of just giving up is the hardest of all, and it normally happens within the first day or two. You must understand, however, that your body has had years of consuming the wrong foods and is racked with toxins that you never thought were there. Even if, you were eating healthy by today's standards, you still have an immense amount of toxins running through your system. We get these toxins from not only the food we eat but, from the air we breathe, and the items we touch throughout the day. Your body will be in a basic "shock" because it will not receive these toxins from food anymore. It will also be flushing these toxins out of your body, and your body will respond by telling you to "just give up." No matter what your mind is telling you, you must persevere through this initial phase and keep up the juicing plan. By the third day and onward, "flame-out" feeling will be replaced with a much more nutritious feeling of "I can't wait for my next glass!" Once you get this feeling, it's smooth sailing through the end.

Once you get past that "flame-out" feeling, you'll begin noticing slight changes. A particular change that most people discover is the restful feeling they wake-up to. The toxins that were in your body at one point are now beginning to decrease, and you'll notice that you'll not only fall asleep faster, you'll require less sleep and wake-up feeling more rested than ever before. This is because you're body is spending less energy digesting and more on rebuilding. Digesting solid foods can require your body to exert up to 30% of your body's total energy level. That leaves the body with only 170% level for rebuilding and working your body. If you have an active lifestyle, then the rebuilding portion of the energy consumption is even less. If your body can't rebuild itself as we're designed to do, then it will begin to break down and not be able to fend off any damages done throughout the day. The result is that we have a much harder time falling asleep, because we are so racked with our bodies trying to rebuild, and we require a much longer time frame for fully sleeping. The only time that our bodies can devote a majority of energy to rebuilding is when we are fully resting. By juicing, our bodies have a chance to begin the rebuilding of our cells throughout the entire day, because there are no solid foods for us to work on digesting.

By allowing our bodies to rebuild on the cellular level, you'll begin to notice that your hair is stronger, fuller and shinier than we could ever imagine. Your fingernails will also go through a tremendous growth spurt and become stronger. Skin becomes smoother, complexion become better, and we gain that natural glow that is normally reserved for only the best of complexions. All of this is possible because you will be removing the toxins and pollutants that we must endure on a daily basis, and from most solid foods we eat.

Lastly, you will begin seeing yourself lose weight. The main reason for this occurrence is due to the increased energy level you'll experience. When you would feel drained and tired, our bodies natural reaction is to sit down and take a "breather." During that time, anything we ate will be stored for later within our bodies. Because we have a tired feeling throughout our day, that stored energy (fat) never gets used and just builds up over time. By having your energy level increased, you are always on the move and your body doesn't feel a need to store anything for later.   What had been stored for later is finally used for energy and you'll notice yourself begin to shed pounds.

As you can see, juicing gives you plenty of reasons to begin your regimen.   Juicing takes only a few minutes a day to set-up, but the results and benefits are lifetime as long as you "maintain" your juicing plans.   Results may vary depending on your particular situation, so, please check with a doctor before you begin your path down a healthier you.

Safe and Healthy Methods of Juicing

Although juicing is a truly healthy way to lose weight, fight off illness, and cleanse the body, there are a few procedures that need to be considered prior to starting your juicing regiment and all through your juicing phase.   If not done in the proper method, juicing has the ability to throw your body into a state of shock and actually be detrimental to your health.   Consider the follow recommendations prior to start of juicing and throughout the entire juicing process.

Before starting any form of juice diet, consult with your doctor.   Be sure your body can handle the effects of juicing.   Juicing will make your body react in a way that it's not accustomed to.   The lack of solid foods will take a toll on an unhealthy body, and if you have any form of irregularities in your immune system, those effects could be terribly damaging.   If this crucial first step is not followed, your health and body could be at stake.   In rare cases, people that have not talked with their doctor prior to beginning a juicing diet have been hospitalized.   The detoxification process that juicing produces will sometime unveil a hidden illness.   Some toxins that we have floating around inside of us tend to suppress certain diseases and illnesses.   Once these are removed, and your body begins to function as nature intended, these diseases surface and could be detrimental to your overall health.   A doctor may request particular test, such as a blood test, if they have any concerns that aren't evident in your current state.

Once your doctor gives you the "all clear to proceed," then you must begin getting your body accustomed to doing without solid foods.   Begin by increasing your liquid intake while reducing your consumption of solid foods.   A good way to do this is to cut your normal meal portion in half beginning two weeks before you plan on kicking off your juicing diet.   If you have a full plate of food and one glass of water, then reduce that portion of food by half and increase your water to two glasses to drink.   The following week reduce your food intake again to only one-fourth a plate while increasing to three or four glasses of drink during your meal.   This will prepare your body to function without the benefits of solid foods.   While doing this, be sure to take a vitamin supplement.   You'll notice that you may feel hungry for the first few days of doing this but, whenever hunger hits, simply drink a glass of water.   During this time, begin cutting down on all caffeine or alcohol drinks.   Caffeine will increase your metabolism and require you to need more energy.   Along with the additional hunger, your blood pressure and heart rate will increase. Alcohol is a key item to stay away from all together prior to, during, and after juicing.   Besides alcohol being a depressant, it also causes dehydration.   You need to keep your liquid levels while juicing, and alcohol will have an adverse reaction to your system.   Besides, caffeine and alcohol are both considered "toxins" and will be removed during the detoxification process.   If an excessive amount of toxins are in your system, it will cause your body to work harder when you actually begin your juicing diet.   Start early by leaving caffeine and alcohol out of your consumption habits and thereby reducing the amount of these toxins prior to juicing.

While juicing will provide your body with many needed nutrients, there are a few needed vitamins and minerals that your body simply can't do without.   One such nutrient that is required for your body to function optimally is protein.   Juicing will provide your body with proteins but, not enough of this needed nutrient.   Protein is found heavily in meats and lightly in fruits and vegetables.   For this reason, it is recommended that you supplement your juicing diet with a protein supplement in pill form.   The best way to keep your digestive system in proper form, juicing experts recommend using the capsule type of pill. You need to take the capsule apart and mix in the protein powder in with your normal juice drink, so your system won't have to try and dissolve the capsule material. Keep in mind that while you're on your juice diet, your system will be accustomed to not having to digest anything solid. This will also speed up the detoxification process within your system.

If you're a newcomer to juicing, begin with fruits and vegetables that you would normally enjoy eating. Some fruits and vegetables aren't too pleasing to the palate and, being new to juicing, you won't care for the taste too much and may quit before you even have a solid chance to enjoy the benefits of juicing. For this reason, keep your juicing variety to a bare minimum. Maybe some strawberries, apples, carrots and other fruits and vegetables that are tasty in their solid form will make a terrific start to developing a "taste" for juicing. Stick with just a few select fruits and vegetables, but mix in both.

Don't just juice fruits that are sweet and tasty. Mix in some other forms of vegetables that you enjoy eating in solid form. Start out small and slow. Let your palate acquire a taste for the other highly beneficial fruits and vegetables such as wheat grass, asparagus, cabbage and the like. Going right to these sometimes awful tasting fruits and vegetables will not be an enjoyable experience. If you elect to begin with a high fruit juice diet, be sure to do so in moderation due to the high sugar levels in sweet fruits. Also, be sure to maintain healthy brushing habits for your teeth because of the high acidic levels in such fruits.

Lastly, even though you may have more energy than you're accustomed to, be sure to use that energy in moderation. Don't participate in any strenuous exercise. Exercise requires protein, carbohydrates and other supplements that will be low in your system. Most of this energy that you'll feel will come from the lack of energy your body normally uses during the digestion process of solid foods.

That means it will be used quickly and leave your muscles, and other organs, hungry for solid foods that it uses as "fuel" after exercising. Even though you'll sleep more peacefully and fully, take it easy during your juicing diet. Many people elect to begin their juicing during a time that doesn't require much activity such as, on vacation, holiday or any extended time away from work. There are a few different juicing diets that are designed with this in mind. More on those later in this book. For now, just remember to take it easy and avoid any strenuous activities.

The Pro's and Con's of Juicing

While the partaking of a solid juice diet has a long list of advantages, there are disadvantages to this outstanding diet plan. Getting back to basics, so to say, juicing will provide our bodies with nutrients and minerals that our advanced everyday lives take away from us. As previously mentioned in this book, our bodies were designed to have a wide variety of fruits and vegetables to choose from. Modern times have limited us to only a select food source due to commercial farming, available land, limited harvest time, and storage methods for our massive population. Juicing is a fantastic way to acquire all the vitamins and minerals that we need to run as efficiently as possible in a short amount of time.

Pro's of Juicing

Juicing with an extensive, yet select choice of high nutrient baring fruits and vegetables will ward off illnesses and diseases of almost every design. Our bodies have a natural defensive mechanism within our genetic make-up that will help us defend against every day, and some not-so every day, illnesses and diseases. We only need to provide the "fuel" to make this happen. Fruit and vegetable juice will provide that much needed "fuel" to make all of this happen. Decades ago, our ancestors were able to get this "fuel" because they grew their own foods (no stores around the corner) and picked it fresh daily or as the crop was ready. Having a large portion of fresh food with their daily meals provided them with all their bodies needed. In today's world, there are many other forms of "work" that we do and rely, on the store, to provide this nutrition for us. Stores are built and run as a form of business to provide for the stores family so, many choices are based on how much money can the store make. This often leaves out many fruits and vegetable minerals we need. Juicing fills the gap in our daily diets.

The time that you're on a juicing diet will cleanse your body of all the toxins that we pick-up under "normal" circumstances. From the air we breathe, to the food we eat, juicing will remove toxins such as pesticides, herbicides, lead, arsenic, amalgam filling, mercury and many more. Even the drugs we take to help our bodies get better will have an adverse reaction over time. One particular organ that suffers the most is the liver. Prescribed and over-the-counter medications can build-up within the liver thus causing it not to work effectively as it was designed to. Juicing will keep the digestive tract simple, and flush out all of these toxins. You'll be left feeling better than ever before because now your body is starting as "fresh" as possible, the way we were designed to.

Many illnesses and diseases are believed to aid in the prevention of or, in some rare occurrences, have been known to cure a wide variety of diseases. Although there is no solid scientific evidence to back up these claims, many avid juicers have a thorough belief in juicing. Some of these diseases and illnesses include:

- ALS (Lou Gehrig's Disease)
- Autism
- Cancer
- Dementia
- Cholesterol Issues
- Migraines
- Pneumonia
- Fibromyalgia
- Bronchitis
- Arthritis

This list is only a short example of some illnesses and diseases that juicing is believed to cure. There are many more, and this is just a short list for demonstration purposes.

A benefit from removing all toxins from your body is a renewed energy level and much more restful sleep. Because the toxins are now removed, your body will not have to work as hard in order to function. Less energy is spent for digestion, breathing, and just moving to more energy can be used in other areas. This benefit can usually be felt within the first few days of undertaking your juicing efforts.

Cleansing your colon is a massive benefit from juicing. Keeping your diet to an unusually simplified liquid form will enable your digestive tract to remove any build-up of solids in your colon and intestines. Once your juicing diet is finished, you will receive a higher level of nutrients from the solid foods that you do eat, thus causing you not to require as much and lose weight. Losing weight will come naturally while juicing even if you aren't on a strict "fat burning" juice diet.

Con's of Juicing

Although juicing has a bevy of benefits, there are a few drawbacks or "con's" to consider. One of the most glaring is the whole premise behind juicing, no solid food intake. For many people, it's hard to fathom not eating, even the slightest, of solids. We've all been taught that we need to enjoy solid foods for fiber and protein. This is a terrifically true statement. We do need both of those, among other advantages that solid foods give us. This is why a juicing diet is only considered "short term." If you permanently stay on it, the juicing diet will harm your body. This is also the reason that many people never even try a juicing plan.

Squeezing the fibers of a fruit or vegetable also gives way to food contamination. Once juice is extracted, E Coli and other bacteria can quickly begin to grow.   The pasteurization process protects the juice from all of the nasty little forms that can get us extremely sick.   By juicing fresh fruits and vegetables yourself, there isn't a pasteurization process, so the juice must be consumed immediately.   Storing this juice for any length of time can slowly turn it from a healthy form of nutrient to an aggressive form of bacteria. Juicing is considered extremely inconvenient and time consuming for this reason.   It takes an extremely determined person that has full discipline to gain the benefits of juicing.   Many people in today's world simply don't have the time for this and, therefore, juicing is not an option open to them.

Another perceived disadvantage of juicing is that you do not gain anything from it in respects to the nutrient level.   Most scientists believe that as soon as you extract the juice from the fibers of fruits and vegetables, exposing the juice to light and air, the vitamins and minerals that would normally be trapped within the fibers are lost. Air and light are the number one enemy of vitamins and minerals. Critics believe you can gain more from fruits and vegetables by simply eating the food in its solid form.   While this may be true, what would have to eat in the solid form would be much greater than you could stomach.   Juicing provides everything you need, nutritionally speaking, in a single serve glass.

Erroneous feelings of excessive energy will be quickly zapped out of your body; you may be left with feeling more fatigued than you felt before.   This is a significant disadvantage of a staunch juicing plan and one that prevents people from staying on it.   Your energy level is a fragile aspect of the human body.   The high level of energy that you feel while eating solid foods is quite different from the high level of energy you feel while juicing.   Energy that you get while juicing is a natural energy that your body produces, not from the food source you consume.   Your body doesn't "naturally" provide this energy.   This energy is "left-over" from the solid foods that you were eating prior to juicing.   Remember, juicing will remove all of the stored solid wastes within your body and the toxins that you've accumulated overtime. Some energy is derived from the left over solids while other energy is produced from the actual toxins.   These two energy sources do not produce much energy.   Feeling energetic comes in small bursts, as those items are removed from your body.   Your energy will quickly be dissipated, and leaving you feeling extremely weak and tired. You must monitor your energy level at all times..   Eating solid foods give you a longer lasting feeling of being energetic.   That's what solid food does; give you "energy to burn."

Weighing Your Options

As you can see, there are some drawbacks to being on a juicing diet.   While these drawbacks are considered, by some individuals, to be too large of an obstacle to overcome, the benefits from juicing are hard to ignore.   Simply weigh the options to see if the "cons" are something that will inevitably prevent you from properly juicing or is it merely something to consider while juicing.

Being properly educated about juicing will make your juicing diet a more pleasurable experience.   One experience that will provide you with lifelong benefits.

Side-Effects of Juicing

If you have ever undertaken a health regime, such as exercise, then you will understand that by changing anything within your normal routine will ultimately lead to side-effects.   Juicing is no different from any other health regime.   Remember the first time you decided to "hit the gym"?   You probably woke-up the next more feeling muscle pain, and stiffness like you never felt before.   Have you ever tried a new diet program?   If you have, then I'm sure you felt some kind of side-effect from it.   Whether it was hunger, fatigue, or cravings, you felt something because you changed your normal eating habits.   This is what you're doing while juice fasting, changing your eating habits.

The above examples are shown to inform you that your body will tend to rebel against you, even though you are only doing it to a healthier body than before juicing.   It still will rebel and throw little tantrums on your mind. You must stick with it, and these side-effects will gradually reduce or stop all together as you get your body used to it.

Some of the side-effects you will, or will not, feel include:

Headaches normally due to the lack of caffeine or alcohol (this is why it was mentioned to reduce these two vices prior to beginning juicing in order to reduce this side-effect)

- Bad Breath
- Lethargy
- Constipation followed by Diarrhea (which if not closely monitored, could lead to serious dehydration)
- Fainting
- Weight Loss
- Vomiting
- Acne (due to drawing out the toxins in your body)
- Hunger

If you have paid attention during the beginnings of this book, you'll understand why your body will be rebelling in this way. Just to ensure you understand why you're body has these side-effects, we'll dive a bit further into each of them.

Headache:

This is predominately due to the lack of caffeine and/or alcohol. Both of these substances are highly addictive to your body, and when there aren't any of these, your body sends signals of pain in order to entice you to succumb to the urge. Do not allow these two toxins to prevail. Another reason you may suffer from a headache during this time is your brain is full of pain notification sensors that when any other part of your body feels pain, it all gathers in your brain. If too many areas feel pain, then your brain goes into somewhat of an overload state and produces a headache. Either way, if you can "grin and bear it," then it is highly suggested you do so. Eventually your body will become accustom to this new form of subsidence you're introducing to it and will stop all pain.

Bad Breath:

This side-effect is fairly common. The reason for this is due to the toxins leaving your body. All toxins produce a smell of some sort. While expelling these out of your body, they literally will make your breath smell awful.

Lethargy:

This goes along with not having the necessary dosage of proteins, sugars, carbohydrates, and fiber that we all require to run efficiently. Have the faith. This too shall pass as long as you understand why it's happening and take extra rest when you need it.

Constipation/Diarrhea:

This side-effect is essentially a double-edged sword against your digestive system. You will first experience dreadful bouts with constipation. This is occurring because your body simply won't know how to respond to the lack of solid foods. It will go into a natural "reserve" mode and try to keep the solids that you have. Once your body learns that no additional solids will be coming into your system, then it will begin to process on a somewhat normal basis. The only problem is that during the "normal" digestive process, there still isn't any solid for it to digest. The fecal matter that we produce is simply the solids that our body doesn't need or doesn't have any nutritional value for us. Our bodies expel this as a waste. The same thing is happening during a juicing diet but, without the presence of solids, the waste is simply liquid. Our digestive system works overtime during juicing, so you will find yourself using the bathroom on a much more frequent basis than prior to your juicing diet. Nothing's wrong with your digestive system, but it won't feel or appear that way. This is one side-effect that you must monitor closely. Because of all the liquid you'll be expelling, you run a severe risk for dehydration. During this time, keep your liquid levels high by either upping the amount of juice you're drinking or consume high volumes of water with your juice.

Fainting:

This can occur simply because you're body has zero energy left. Many times, people that don't take additional rest and simply goes about their normal daily activities will suffer from this side-effect. This is easily overcome by simply slowing down, but many people find it hard to slow down to the extent that may be required. Be sure to get an ample amount of rest and limit yourself to the kind of activities you perform.

Weight Loss:

Simply put, you have no excess solids in your system, so you will naturally lose weight. Unless you are severely underweight, this side-effect is often welcomed by individuals that go on a juice diet.

Vomiting:

Once again, your body will be throwing a temper tantrum because you are now removing particular foods from your diet. The way it reacts is by simply expelling what it doesn't want. A few other reasons that this may occur is by consuming juices that may have been stored for too long or not stored properly. Remember, juice is a bastion for parasites and bacteria. All they need to grow is a little time and temperature in order to grow by the thousands quickly. Reduce your risk of vomiting due to this by drinking only fresh from the fruit or vegetable juice.   Try not to store it and if you do, store it in an air-tight, dark container for a decidedly limited time in a refrigerated place.   Remember, the three basic elements for bacteria and parasites to thrive in are air, light and warm temperatures.   Lastly, one of the most common of all reasons for vomiting is simply because your palate doesn't like the taste of the juice you're drinking.   Mix it up and try different flavors.   Begin first with fruits and vegetables that you genuinely enjoy in their solid form.   Once you get your body and palate use to drinking juice, then you can begin slowly mixing in small amounts of the more beneficial, but less tasty, juices.

Acne:

This side-effect goes right along with the bad breath.   Your skin is a living organ, even though many of us don't think of it as one. It is also plagued with toxins on a daily basis.   Juicing will remove toxins from your skin, and they will be expelled in the form of acne. As your juicing diet goes on, you'll begin to see less acne because the toxins are slowly being dwindled down.

Hunger:

This is a clear side-effect that everyone will already understand. Eating no solid foods equals hunger in the beginning stages.   When you feel like you simply can't stand it anymore, just drink more juice or water, and your hunger pains will go away.

Regardless of how you may feel about getting through any of these side-effects, if they become too serious, please go to your doctor or hospital.   Inform them that you are on a juicing diet, so they can take the necessary actions to ensure your health.   If these side-effects become too serious, or last for several days, they can cause serious injury.   Seek medical attention immediately.

Know Your Juice

Now that, you know and understand the basics of a juicing diet, you need to understand what a particular fruit and vegetable juice will provide. There are many other fruits and vegetables to explore, but this short listing of the most common "beginner" juices will demonstrate the nutrients that juicing will give you.

Orange:

Maybe one of the most common fruit juices, orange juice will provide you with a multitude of benefits.   One of the known benefits is the rich amount of Vitamin C that is throughout the orange.   The lesser known nutrients are the amount of antioxidants that it contains. When these two nutrients combine, they flood your muscles, bones, skin and blood with the building blocks they need to grow and get stronger.   Be sure to mix in a bit of orange juice in with your daily juice consumption.

Apple:

Apple juice is one of the best fruits to keep your heart pumping as optimally as possible.   The vast amount of phytonutrients that it contains will drastically reduce the amount of crude cholesterol in your body.   The high amount of fiber and Vitamin C it contains will benefit muscle and bone growth along with giving your skin a healthy appearance.   The adage of "An apple a day keeps the doctor away" got its start simply from the fact that an apple keeps your heart healthy by combating levels of unhealthy cholesterol.

Grape:

A long-time choice for many children, grape juice is much more than just a refreshing juice. The blend of sweet and sour that it provides delights our palates, which makes it number one on almost any persons list of juices. The robust levels of antioxidants maintain our cardiovascular system and lowers blood pressure. All the taste with a multitude of essential health benefits keeps this form of fruit juice on all juicing diet lists.

Tomato:

The phytonutrients, lycopene and beta-carotene, that tomato juice provide are powerful antioxidants to ward off any toxins that your body may harbor. The Vitamin E levels in tomato juice are often overlooked when some individuals pick what juice to mix into their juicing diets. Vitamin E provides the essential nutrients to your skin to maintain a healthy appearance. Two other benefits that tomato juice will give you are an increased immune system to combat illnesses along with lowered blood pressure for a healthier heart.

Carrot:

An often missed "super" vegetable, carrot juice is loaded with vitamins and minerals that the metabolism in the body craves. It has Vitamin A, B Vitamins, chlorine, iron, calcium, sodium magnesium and sulfur. All of these vitamins and minerals combine to flood your metabolism system with nutrients to have your body working on the highest level possible. Be sure to add a little carrot juice, at the minimum, daily to keep your body in tip-top shape.

Strawberry:

One of the best tasting fruits to fight cancer, strawberry juice has a high level of ellagic acid that reduces the risk of cancer cells forming. The iron that is hidden inside this tasty fruit has been shown to produce red blood cells which also aids in cancer prevention. The levels of potassium it contains control the risk of having high blood pressure. Maintaining your blood pressure will keep your heart healthy for years to come.

Acai Berry:

While we are on the topic of fighting cancer, the Acai Berry is well-known throughout the world as being the new superfood to fight off, prevent, and in rare occurrences, cure cancer. Found in the deep recesses of the rain forest, the Acai Berry can now be found in most large supermarkets. Truly, it's one of the world's best cancer prevention juices available.

Black Cherry:

While being well-known for its high levels of antioxidants, the Vitamin C they contain can only be considered worthwhile if taken in large amounts. This little cherry is considered to be one of the best to drink after a hard exercise routine. The nutrients that it holds reduce muscle inflammation that may occur after a vigorous workout. Muscles naturally produce lactic acid inside of them during exercise, and this acid builds up to produce swelling, which in turn causes muscle aches and pains. The nutrients inside of the black cherry reduce this lactic acid which prevents the muscles from swelling and causing pain. It is a great after work-out juice to consume even while, not on a juicing diet. Remember one of the rules of juicing. Do not partake in vigorous workouts while juicing. Mix in this juice only for flavor, antioxidants and small amounts of Vitamin C. Keep juicing this marvelous little fruit even after your juicing diet has ended.

Blueberry:

Every food group seems to have its own form of "brain food." In reference to the fruit food group, blueberries are considered the "brain food." The high levels of antioxidants, vitamins and fiber all have massive benefits to heal body cells and brain inflammation that happens as we get older. Blueberries are natures own "Fountain of Youth."

Pomegranate:

While not on many lists due to the sometimes considered bitter taste, the pomegranate is considered to be the best fruit available for antioxidants due to the various antioxidants it holds. Various antioxidants have been well-known to be the key to fighting cancer and premature aging. The pomegranate has an immense variety of these antioxidants. For this reason, it comes in second to the Acai Berry for its cancer fighting abilities. Pomegranate juice is ranked number one amongst all other forms of juice for its anti-aging properties.

Grapefruit:

We have heard of grapefruit juice benefit to lose weight. However, grapefruit juice has many lesser known benefits. It has been known to fight illnesses, cancer, fatigue, eye problems, skin disorders and a bevy of other problems that our bodies may suffer from. It has a multitude of nutrients such as Vitamin, B complexes, Vitamin E, Vitamin K, Calcium, Folic Acid, Potassium, Phosphorus and a host of phytonutrients such as Flavonoids, Liminoids and Lycopene. As you can see, the grapefruit has much more to offer the human body besides keeping our weight manageable.

Cabbage:

When thinking of juicing vegetables, cabbage is probably the last one you'd think of squeezing the juice from. If you don't juice cabbage, you're missing out on one of the most beneficial vegetables for juicing. Cabbage juice is loaded with vital phytonutrients that our bodies thrive upon. Phytonutrients such as sulforaphane will produce enzymes for detoxification and the production of Glutathione, which is a vital enzyme for liver detoxification. Red cabbage offers a wider variety of phytonutrients primarily because of the red color of the cabbage. Any vegetable that is red in color has an added phytonutrient called anthocyanin. Anthocyanin is an antioxidant that has been proven to aid in the protection of brain cells, which can help in the prevention of Alzheimer's. Cabbage juice has also been proven to build muscle fibers, strengthen the eyes and cleanse the blood. The iron and sulfur content in fresh, raw cabbage juice has further been proven to heal ulcers and fight fungal infections. Fresh, raw cabbage juice is certainly a form of juice that needs to be included in any juicing diet plan.

Wheatgrass:

Being the last to be included on this list of common fruits and vegetables, wheatgrass juice is known as the "do-it-all" form of juice. It helps in all areas of the body and when mixed with other juices, has no taste. It detoxifies all parts of the body, helps maintain weight, balances the pH in your body, and produces red blood cells. It is unbelievably similar to our own blood in what it can offer our bodies. Definitely a juice to have in your juicing arsenal.

This is only a short list of the most common and beneficial juices that you need to know. There are many others available for you to take full advantage of. Almost any fruit or vegetable that you can imagine will be loaded, with essential vitamins and minerals, to keep your body in the utmost of shape. Mix and match different juices depending on your personal taste preferences and your own personal health goals. Regardless of what your health aspirations may be, there will be a juice to get your body on the pathway of living a healthy lifestyle.

Juicing for Weight Loss

Many people begin their path on a juicing diet for one basic task, to lose weight. Along the way, they discover that juicing actually has many other healthy benefits besides just for weight loss. However, losing weight is what first sparked their interest in juicing diets. If you fall into this category of juicers, then this section of the book is just for you.

When undertaking a juice diet for weight loss, you must first understand that there is a variety of different fruits and vegetables for you to choose from. There is not just one single fruit or vegetable that you can lose weight with. The selection is on a grand scale and will aid in your sticking to your juicing plan because of the variety. Too often, many individuals simply give up or "cheat" during their weight loss plan because they become bored with what they are required to eat to achieve their goal. When dieting with juice, becoming bored with your diet can quickly be overcome by mixing up your meal plan.

Along that though process, keep in mind that there isn't a particular food group you need to consume. You can pick an all fruit juicing diet, an all vegetable juicing diet or a combination of both. Foods from each group have their own benefits, in respects to losing weight. However, when looking for the benefit of fiber, buying fruit juice or juicing your own fruits and vegetables will not give you the recommended daily allowance of fiber. Processed fruit juice or fresh fruit juice removes a tremendous amount of fiber from the fruit or vegetable. For this reason, it is recommended that you do not juice your fruit or vegetable. Instead, drop a clean, whole fruit or vegetable in a blender until liquefied.   This will keep all of the fiber that your selected food has, and you will not lose any of the fiber benefits from that food.

Typical Vegetables for Weight Loss

An all vegetable juice diet, when mixed in a blender, the juice keeps its high fiber content and is an effective way to lose the dreaded hunger pains and potential dehydration.   Vegetables are high in fiber and water content which provides a long lasting feeling of fullness. Fiber requires your body to use more energy to process and requires more time to process. The full feeling you will get from the fiber will last for extended periods of time.   The water content within the vegetables will ward aid in the prevention of dehydration that often occurs during a weight loss diet.

Spinach:

Spinach has been a long-time staple for any vegan diet. It has a high amount of fiber and doesn't cause the body to retain water, thus limiting the bloated feeling.   The amount of Vitamin A, Vitamin C, Vitamin E, Vitamin K, Thiamin, Riboflavin, Calcium, Iron, Potassium, Manganese, Vitamin B6, Folate, Magnesium, Phosphorous, and Copper is second to none.   All of these vital nutrients benefit our bodies in a number of ways.

Collard Greens:

This delightful vegetable is loaded with proteins and amino acids while having a low glycemic index.   Having vitamins like Vitamin A, Vitamin C, Vitamin E, Vitamin K, Riboflavin, Folate, Manganese, Calcium, and Vitamin B6, collard greens causing the body to burn stored amounts of fat in the form of energy.

Brussel Sprouts:

While having almost all the added benefits of cabbage, brussel sprouts won't produce gaseous formations within your body. Brussel sprouts are low-calorie and low in fat; it has nutrients like Vitamin A, Vitamin C, Vitamin K, Vitamin B6, folate, potassium, thiamin and manganese. Being a low-fat, low-calorie food while providing all the above mentioned nutrients, it is considered to be a complete vegetable juice to mix into your normal weight loss juicing diet.

Broccoli:

It has as significant source of carbohydrates and protein, broccoli is made up of 60% carbohydrates and 40% proteins. The carbohydrate complex of broccoli is intense enough to require the body to take additional time in the digestion process, warding off the dreaded hunger pains. The massive carbohydrate content in broccoli is slow-releasing so you'll have ample energy to get through your day. Broccoli contains vital minerals and vitamins such as Iron, Calcium, Pantothenic Acid, Thiamin, Selenium, Phosphorous, Magnesium, Riboflavin, and Vitamin E. It is considered by many to be the single-most valuable vegetable to be included in any weight loss juicing diet.

Beans:

Having an exorbitant amount of protein and dietary fibers, the bean is quite pleasing to your palate, even when eaten raw or as a juice. Being low in fat and high in protein and fiber make them the perfect partner in your weight loss goals.

Carrots:

Having the same fiber and protein amounts as the above mentioned beans, carrots also have a rich content of Vitamin A,

Vitamin C, Vitamin K and other necessary minerals. Among all the above mentioned benefits, carrot juice is a naturally refreshing and filling juice to have on a regular basis.

Typical Fruits for Weight Loss

Typically, you will want to stay away from most fruit juices during your weight loss undertakings. Fruit juice is high in sugars and calories and will be burned as energy by your body instead of your body using the stored fat that you have.

However, there are a select few fruits that you can safely juice that will promote weight loss, have low sugar levels, and are low in calories. Some of the listed fruits will give you the energy that you need during your typical day and will burn away that unwanted fat instead of just burning the energy away from the juice.

Cranberry:

Besides being a refreshing juice drink choice, cranberry juice contains many beneficial nutrients to aid in combating your weight. Being immensely high in Vitamin C, cranberry juice also has an absorbent amount of antioxidants. These antioxidants help maintain your urinary tract and will prevent, or in some occurrences, cure E Coli infections within your bladder. Cranberry juice can be mixed, with other fruits or vegetables, to enhance your health while detoxifying your body.

Mango:

This tropical fruit contains an exceptionally high level of antioxidants which will help in the prevention of a variety of different cancers. The juice from a mango has the added benefit of cleansing your bloodstream from toxins, which will lead to a much improved circulatory system.   The mango is also a healthy choice for detoxification of your kidneys.   It will keep the kidneys functioning well.   Like many other fruits on this list, the mango mixes extremely well with other fruits.   The sweetness of the mango should be mixed with fruits only, the taste differences between the mango and most vegetables may leave you with an unusual taste.

Pears:

Pear juice may be considered one of the most well-balanced fruit juices available to us.   Besides its stand alone consummate taste, when mixed with other fruit juices, pear juice explodes your palate with a variety of exciting flavors.   The high levels of Potassium, Magnesium, Phosphorous, Vitamin C, and Calcium round out this exciting fruit.   Be sure to have pears handy at all times during your weight loss diet.   This fruit will not disappoint you.

Oranges:

Orange juice has been known, for a long time, to be a healthy fruit drink for our bodies.   The amount of the antioxidant, Flavonoid, is only shadowed by the high levels of Vitamin C this fruit holds within its thick outer skin.   Vitamin C has been well-known for many decades to be the number one fighter against illnesses by strengthening the immune system.   The antioxidant, Flavonoid, has been verified to increase blood flow throughout your circulatory system, including your heart.   This juice will not be too difficult to drink either.   The perfect, refreshing taste it holds has been welcomed by many people for many years.

Purple Grapes:

The first and foremost benefit to drinking purple grape juice is the protection of brain cells.   It has been discovered that memory improves drastically by drinking the purple grape.   This research has been proven to help aid in the prevention of the memory crippling disease, Alzheimer's. The high levels of antioxidants this little grape holds have further been proven to fight against a variety of diseases. As with any fruit juice, purple grape juice is most beneficial in its unprocessed state and not bought from the store and drank immediately after liquefying.

Pomegranate:

Another delightfully refreshing juice, pomegranate juice has almost every antioxidant known to man hidden inside it. Long known by health experts, pomegranate juice is extremely healthy for the heart and circulatory system. Due to the high levels of antioxidants in it, pomegranate juice is also well-known for fighting almost any form of cancer.

Blueberries:

As with any blue or purple colored fruit, blueberries hold a high-level of antioxidants to fight against a variety of diseases. One lesser known nutrient that blueberries hold is Vitamin C and high fiber levels. Both of these nutrients are the building blocks to a healthy body. The low caloric value that this exceptional fruit has makes it an excellent fruit to have for your weight loss diet.

Concord Grapes:

As you can see from its coloring, the concord grape holds an immense level of antioxidants. These antioxidants produce nitric oxide that increases the size of blood vessels and arteries. The result is a much lower blood pressure and a decidedly healthy heart. Concord grape juice is truly a heart healthy choice.

Does Juicing Work For Weight Loss?

This is a common question for many new juicers. Simply put, juicing does work. It will help you in your efforts to lower your weight more effectively than any other diet you've been on. However, with that being said, there is a particular way that you must juice your fruits or vegetables in regards to losing weight.

The fruit or vegetable must be blended in a blender as to keep the necessary fiber your body needs in order for weight loss to happen. Fiber is an indispensable component in fruits and vegetables. Many vitamins and minerals are stored in the fiber of the fruit or vegetable, and if this is removed during the normal juicing process, all of those additional vitamins and minerals will be lost.

When juicing for weight loss, the fiber helps to keep you satisfied for longer amounts of time. Your body will require a longer period of time to process and digest the fiber, so you will not feel hungry for longer durations in comparison to drinking just the juice. The fiber in the fruit or vegetable in your juicing choice will also help to maintain your insulin levels. Your body will burn the stored fat reserve instead of the insulin from the juice, if you maintain a normal insulin level within your body. By doing this, it becomes a more effective form for you to lose weight.

So, in conclusion, juicing only works for weight loss if done properly. Be sure to puree your fruit or vegetable choice in a blender to gain all the added benefits of the fiber nutrient. With regard to which food group to choose from when trying to lose unwanted pounds, many experts agree that the vegetable food group is the best method. Fruit has higher sugar levels than vegetables do, so the body will burn the calories from the sugar before it burns calories from stored fat reserves. That's not to say simply do an all vegetable juicing regime. There are many benefits to fruit juice that you will also receive. Health experts all have laid testimony stating that the best method to lose weight from juicing is a balanced meal plan from both food groups.

What Results to Expect

The results that you can expect while on a juicing diet will depend on your level of commitment to the diet. Typical results have shown to be anywhere from 3 to 4 pounds per day for the first week. This is mostly water weight that you will be losing but, you will still notice the amount on your scale. From that point forward, it will level off to be around 1 to 2 pounds per day for the duration of the diet. Research studies have shown that individuals have lost on the average of 30 pounds while on a 30 day juice diet. Theoretically speaking, you could lose as much as your whole body mass and die from starvation if you decide to stay permanently on a juice diet.

While juice diets are excellent for short term, it is not recommended to be a permanent food plan. Our bodies need more than what an all juice diet will give us. Giving your body a break every now and then is undeniably a splendid idea to think about.

Digesting the normal solid foods that we eat gives us much of what our bodies are required to have, but is seriously taxing on our digestive system. On average, it takes around 5 hours for our bodies to digest solid foods and just 15 minutes for our bodies to digest or absorb all of the nutrients we need from juice. Studies have shown that our bodies require must less energy to digest juice, while we require much more energy for solid food digestion. The time we spend on an all juice diet gives our system time to relax and flush out all of the toxins that we have. Eating fast foods or processed foods like much of us normally do puts an abundance of pollutants in our organs. A juice diet will flush all of these pollutants out and leave us with a great feeling.

By giving our bodies a break and requiring less energy toward digestion, there is more energy to be spent on losing those unwanted pounds. While juice gives us much of the nutrients we need, the one nutrient that is not present is protein. When on a juice diet, our bodies still use protein during our normal activities, but it uses the stored protein we have in our fat reserves. By our bodies seeking out protein in this form, it uses that fat thus making you lose weight.

Although a juice diet will get you results quickly, simply doing it to revisit your old eating habits is not a permanent solution.   Losing weight is a life changing experience.   An experience that you must take with you for years to come.   Juice diets will get you to your goal weight, but it is up to you to remain there.   Even after your initial juice diet has ended, continuing a one-day juice diet once a week or once a month is a fantastic way to keep those unwanted pounds permanently off.   You'll feel terrific, have more energy, and gain confidence from your experience.

Juicing the Toxins Out

Besides just juicing for weight loss, many have undertaken juice fasting to rid their bodies of pollutants and toxins from the everyday foods we all eat.   Even if, you eat healthy from the store, you'll still have an amount of toxins coursing through your body. These toxins are from the process foods we all purchase.   Unless you strictly purchase your foods from a whole foods store, or grow your own food, you will have pollutants from process foods in your system that need to be flushed out from time to time.

If you are wondering why you need to remove these toxins if you are otherwise feeling healthy, think of how you would feel if you could actually absorb all of the nutrients that the food you eat offer. Over time, even if you eat "healthy", you will have a buildup of solids that are acting like a barrier between your body and the healthy food you're eating.   Vital nutrients are simply being expelled from your body as waste, and you're only receiving around 10% of the nutrient content that food has in it.   Removing this barrier of solids from the digestive system will allow your body to absorb around 90% of the nutritional value of whatever food you're consuming.

The average person is already not receiving the recommended daily allowances of nutritional value from a variety of foods.   This already puts your body behind on nutrients.   If these solids that have built-up in your system remain in place, then you are receiving a drastically smaller amount of vital nutrients to keep you healthy.   Put yourself on a regular pattern for juicing and remove these solids and regain all of what you have lost.   The final result will leave you feeling much more energetic, a more manageable body weight, and able to ward off a number of illnesses or diseases.

Kidney

Kidneys normally take the brunt of any toxins that you may consume from the foods you eat.   It is the body's filtration system that all things ingested must pass through.   As we eat processed foods or fast foods that are loaded with toxins, the kidneys job is to remove as much of these bad items that it can.   The stress that the kidneys go through is tremendous, and they need to have a break from time to time and be cleansed.   A juice diet will wash much of that away and leave the kidneys in a much healthier state.

Good fruits to juice to cleanse your kidneys are lemons, cranberries, apples, pineapples, watermelons and a large majority of other citrus fruits.   Vegetables to consider for cleaning your kidneys are foods such as cucumbers, asparagus, carrots and cabbage.   There are a couple of herbs you can throw in with the vegetable drink to enhance the taste.   Those herbs are parsley and mint; both are also advantageous for the kidneys.   Lastly, be sure to drink plenty of purified or filtered water.   The recommended intake of this kind of water is 8 8oz glasses at a minimum.   Try to shoot for any number greater than that.   Your kidneys will thank you for it.

Liver

The liver controls many functions of your body.   From secreting enzymes for digestion to breaking down toxins in your blood, the liver is the largest internal organ your body has.   It is also the first organ to be considered for cleaning purposes for this reason.   If your liver isn't functioning at an optimal level, everything you eat or drink doesn't get processed in the way it should be processed, and you will not receive all nutrients from your food or, even worse, get sick.

Some good foods to consider for detoxifying your liver should be tomatoes, cucumbers, beet juice, garlic, and papayas.   Mix these in any combination you want, and you'll have a clean and well functioning liver.

Colon

The colon is often referred to as the bodies trash can.   This is where a large majority of your bodies waste is expelled from the system.   Over time, this waste can build-up and cause severe trauma to your digestive system in the form of constipation, diarrhea, gas, and a number of other conditions.   It also can contribute to not allowing the needed nutrients to be absorbed into your blood stream.   A thick fecal barrier can be formed which will prevent your body from absorbing all of the potential nutrients of the foods you eat. Removing this barrier by performing a colon cleansing will enable your digestive system to perform in the way it was designed to.

Vegetables you should eat to cleanse your colon include items such as lettuce, wheatgrass, carrots, broccoli, and celery.   Good fruits to mix into your diet are apples, cranberries, grapefruits, orange, and pineapples.   Try to limit yourself on citrus fruits as they have a tendency to slow down your digestive system.

Skin

While many people don't think of their skin this way, skin is an organ.   One that is bombarded with pollutants and toxins not only from the inside, but from the outside also.   For this reason, when you're detoxifying your body, be sure to think of your skin.

Acne, psoriasis, paleness, chaffing, and a number of other skin conditions can all be linked back to toxins and pollutants.   When you eat a processed or fast food, the toxins not only harm your inside organs, but your skin from the inside to the outside.   Sunshine can be detrimental to your skin health as well as air pollution.   Probably the most of all organs that will succumb to the harshness of toxins, the skin will be the first noticeable organ to be polluted.

Skin detoxification foods include items such as apples, leafy greens, pumpkin, watercress, pears, cucumber, carrots, and grapes. Good herbs to cleanse your skin are calendula, dandelion, evening primrose oil, fennel, and milk thistle.

Lung

Often overlooked, the lung is a crucial organ that we simply cannot live without. It gives us life by inhaling the air that we need to survive. Remarkably, individuals often miss this hugely valuable organ during their detoxification program.

Lungs basically seek-out toxins and pollutants. Although not intentionally, toxins and pollutants found in the air we breathe are drawn into the lungs. This happens every day of our lives for we need to breath in order to live. A rather serious organ to detoxify once you think about it.

Food to consider juicing when detoxifying your lungs would include items such as spinach, squash, slippery elm, wild cherry bark, cinnamon, onions, beets, oranges, and apples.

Gallbladder

The gallbladder is an organ that we only miss if it has been removed. The effects of not having a gallbladder vary dependent on a person's diet. They can range from bloating to diarrhea and always include massive stomach discomfort.

The gallbladder's function is to be a storage vessel for bile that the liver produces. During the digestion process, the gallbladder will squirt a bit of this bile into our system to aid in digestion of food

When the gallbladder isn't functioning properly, or isn't present to accept the bile from the liver, the bile then passes through the digestive tract which results in the above mentioned symptoms. If the gallbladder becomes too toxic, then it produces gallstones that are essentially balls of toxic residue that the gallbladder has formed and must be released. Gallstones are immensely painful, and anyone that has had them would recommend simply to avoid them by detoxifying your gallbladder.

Gallbladder friendly foods to cleanse with include carrots, ginger root, apples, cabbage, garlic, chives, mint, parsley, and basil.

Pancreas

In a nutshell, the pancreas controls both the digestive system as well as the endocrine system. When this organ gets too many toxins in it, and doesn't perform effectively, our insulin and hormone levels will become erratic. Fluctuating insulin will lead to diabetes while unbalanced hormones can lead to a multitude of medical problems. Keeping this vital organ in the utmost of condition is extremely pertinent to the rest of the bodies overall health.

There are many specialty stores that sell pre-made pancreas flushing supplements. Another option is making your own out of a select few herbs such as comfrey root, devil's club, huckleberry, juniper berries, golden seal root, and a host of others. For this reason, it is recommended not to make your own pancreatic cleansing drink. Undertaking a solid overall body cleanse and supplementing with the pre-made pancreatic cleanse is the best option. Be sure to drink 7 to 10 glasses of water a day while taking these supplements. Water will flush the toxins out of the pancreas quicker and leave it in a much better state.

Blood

Blood is the liquid form of life. Without it, none of our organs would function, and we would simply die. The blood is the unwilling carrier of all toxins and pollutants.   Considering that everything we do, from breathing the air to touching with our hands, can be absorbed into our bloodstream and carried to vital organs; it would only be the wise choice to cleanse our blood.   Outside pollutants can act in a variety of ways to our blood, so it is difficult to say exactly how toxins will react with a particular person's blood. From breaking down individual blood cells to morphing those cells into something devilishly different than what it was designed to do, toxins wreck havoc on our bloodstream.   Cleansing the blood will regain the efficiency of what our blood was meant to do, carry oxygen throughout the body.

People must utilize the nutrients found in juices such as carrots, beets, lemon, and any leafy green juices, to cleanse the blood. The green color means that the juice has chlorophyll.   Chlorophyll is an essential nutrient in blood cleansing because it builds up the important nutrients within the cells and inhibits cell damage due to the suns radiation.   Particular juices that have plenty of chlorophyll stored in them are alfalfa, barley and wheatgrass.

Full Body Assault

Naturally, you now have a basic roadmap to all of your vital organs.   Combining all of these together with similar fruits and vegetables will give you an overall "full body cleanse" that you may be seeking.   The one side note that you must adhere to is to perform the colon cleanse first.   As experts have stated, a full-body cleanse first starts with the colon.

The cleansing process will expel the toxins and pollutants from your body, which means that crummy stuff has to go somewhere, if it's to be removed from your body.   In other words, you will be going to the bathroom a lot during your cleansing process.   Having your colon in shape to handle all of this above average usage will keep the process of cleansing going smoothly, and keep you in better health along the way.   If your colon isn't in optimal performance, then the toxins that are trapped inside can back-up in your system and cause significant illness in particular areas of your body.   Keeping your colon clean and flowing well will prevent this from happening.

Once your colon is effectively working, then you can begin your total body cleansing.   Lay out a variety of different organ specific recipes.   You'll soon notice that there are several fruits and vegetables that you can use to cover several organs at once.   This will enable you not to worry about doing individual cleansing and stay on a juice diet for unnecessary lengths of time.

Juicing for Health

Many times, people turn to juicing simply to overcome or prevent a particular illness or disease.   This has been performed throughout the ages.   The first recorded fast came in the form of natural water fasting where the individual going on a fast would drink only water.   During this recorded time, it was done not only to aid in fighting illness, but for religious reasons.   We've come a long way since that time and now understand that fasting on just water is seriously detrimental to our health.   Research on a variety of fruits and vegetables has concluded that there is much to be gained from juicing these foods.

Diabetes

Diabetes has become all too common in today's world. Unfortunately, diabetes is predominately due to the diet that we eat. The good news out of this is that it is our diet, and we can somewhat control how our bodies react by changing our diets.   The basic dysfunction that leads to diabetes is our system not being able to break down insulin to normal levels.   This will produce spikes of high sugar levels.   These spikes are detrimental to the body's health and must be regulated through diet and medicine.   It's an ongoing battle of monitoring the bloods sugar levels and adjusting diet and medicine for the diabetes sufferer that they must deal with their entire life.

Juicing particular vegetables can regain some control in this battle. While juicing fruits are not recommended due to the high sugar content, above ground vegetables are unusually low in sugar content and considered safe for diabetes sufferers. As a general rule, below ground vegetables such as carrots, potatoes, and beets have almost as must sugar content as fruits do, above ground vegetables such as cabbage, lettuce, and tomatoes have remarkably little to no sugar content. Staying with this general rule-of-thumb will provide all the benefits of juicing for diabetes sufferers as though they never had the dreaded condition.

Cancer Prevention

The causes of cancer are many, but prevention of cancer is fairly straightforward to do. Just increase your intake of fruits and vegetables. It's that simple. Juicing allows you to consume enormous amounts of fruits and vegetables in a single glass. You may receive one to three servings of your daily intake of fruits and vegetables all within on juicing meal. This enables the body to begin repairing itself from all of the "unhealthy" eating you've done in the past. Juicing is the best method for your body to absorb as much nutrition as possible in a short amount of time. Your body will act like a sponge and suck all of the nutrients directly into your bloodstream where the repairs will begin immediately.

All people are born with cancer. Cancer is simply a deformed cell that behaves in a strange way. It is not welcomed by the rest of your body and white blood cells consistently attack it to kill it and remove the cancerous cell. When cancer forms in the way we all understand someone to have cancer, this means that person's body has simply run out of white blood cells, and the cancer cells are now outnumbering them. Once this happens, cancer invades all parts of our body and begins destroying vital organs. Keeping your white blood cells high in volumes will prevent the cancer from overwhelming your body.

Fruit and vegetables are the best way to keep needed nutrients flowing into your blood. These nutrients build more white blood cells and thus, keeping us healthy. Foods that are high in carotenoids, such as carrots will drastically change your cancer risk to low or non-existent levels. Also, mix in some juices that contain lycophene. Lycophene is an antioxidant and can be found in a number of fruits from strawberries to watermelons. Lastly, look for food choices that are high in fiber and Vitamin E. If you are strictly juicing for cancer prevention or cure, then it would be wise to not just juice your fruits and vegetables. Puree them in a blender as to retain all of the natural fiber they have to offer. Fiber is a fantastic way to ward off cancer cells.

Digestive Disorders

Juicing in general will provide you with digestion relief. The basic of juicing is that your body will not require the time nor energy to digest juice compared to digesting solid foods. As mentioned previously, it takes approximately 5 hours for your body to digest any solid food while it only takes 15 minutes for it to digest juice. The amount of energy it uses is tremendously less than that of solid foods, so your body gets a break to make self repairs. Oftentimes after juicing, people that have had digestive disorders report that they are quite cured of whatever digestive ailment befell them. Sometimes all the body needs is a slight break in order for it to fix itself. Other times, it may be something more serious that may require a visit to your doctor.

A few nutritious foods to juice and give your body a rest are cabbage, papaya, pineapple, and apples. These are only a select few of the best that will cover whatever your digestive disorder may be and is a superb starting point to allow your body to have a digestive rest.

Energy

As mentioned throughout this book, juicing fruits and vegetables will provide you with ample energy. While, on a juicing diet, you may notice times of feeling lethargic and unmotivated. These are times that your body is cleansing itself of all the toxins. Shortly thereafter, you may have a burst of energy like you've never had before. This is due to the fact that, because the toxins are removed, your body is finally receiving the nutrients it hungers for. By juicing regularly, this barrier of toxins will not be able to build itself up and form a wall between your body and the nutritional value that the juice holds.

However, there are a few specific fruits and vegetables that will give you that little extra burst of energy you may be seeking. They include foods such as carrots, parsley, and spinach. Fruit and vegetable juice contain complex B Vitamins, Potassium and Magnesium. All of these nutrients are the building blocks to increased energy and stamina levels. After a few days of juicing in this fashion, you should notice that you've gained energy and stamina. Keep juicing for additional energy and stamina throughout the year, even while, not on a juice diet. The changes in your energy and stamina levels will be markedly increased the longer you keep drinking the juice.

Anti-Aging and Longevity

As a general rule, juicing will add quality years to your life and keep you looking younger than you looked prior to juicing. All of this is from the benefits of simply removing the toxins and pollutants from your body while giving you all the nutrients your body is required to have. In today's world of "quick and easy", the nutritional value of our food has dropped drastically. This drop in nutrients has left our bodies in a state of despair. It is so common today that the regular person doesn't even realize just how unhealthy they actually are. If they were to begin a juicing diet, they would clearly see the positive changes their bodies will undergo simply from eating in the way we were designed to eat. Not many people grow their own food anymore. Supermarkets fill that need for us.

Processed foods have their advantages and disadvantages. One notable advantage from processed food is the risk of parasites that may grow from improperly stored fresh food, a common problem in earlier times. The disadvantage of having processed food is the lessening of needed nutrients. By means of processing the food for health concerns, it's a double-edged sword that removes most of the nutritional value the food once had.

Juicing fresh fruits and vegetables regains this loss and our bodies thank us for it by not only feeling young again, but looking young. Our skin will glow, wrinkles will fade, and joints will feel fabulous once again.

While juicing anything will turn the hands of time back, juicing particular fruits and vegetables high in antioxidants, phytonutrients and enzymes will reap the largest of rewards for your efforts. Some of the foods that are high in all of these nutrients are fresh water blue algae, wheatgrass, goji berry, maca, bee pollen, a variety of sea vegetables such as seaweed, wakame and kelp, and sprouts of all kinds are all known as "Superfoods" because they do contain vast amounts of nutrients for our bodies. While not terribly pleasing to the palate, be sure to mix in some or all of these varieties of Superfoods into your normal juicing regimen. The changes should be felt within a matter of a couple of short weeks.

Tips for Success

No matter how impressive your juicing diet plan may be, it will only work as well as you want it to. If you have a tendency to "cheat" during diets, then juicing will not give you all of the noticeable differences you may otherwise have. The best way to ensure your success while on a juicing diet is to devise a plan and stick to it. If you happen to "fall off the wagon," don't just give up. Jump right back on your juicing diet. Eventually, you will be able to get through the entire plan regardless of how long it may be.

Plan Ahead

Whether you decide to undergo a 1, 3, 5, 15 or even 30 day juicing diet, a plan must be made prior to your undertaking it. If you are a new juicer, then simply try to get through a 1 day plan. If that may seem a bit too much for you, back it down to just mixing in a juice meal instead of your normal meal. Write down the reasons why you want to do a juice diet. What changes you want to make to your health. Is it for an illness? Then write down the people you care about that would like to have you around for many years. Is it for a weight loss goal? Then write down the reason why you want to lose weight and the weight you want to reach. Revisit this list during times of weakness to reinforce your determination and give you the strength you will need to endure this life changing diet. When everything is said and done, you will be thankful that you decided to give juicing a try. You may even notice such a drastic change in your health; you may want to continue mixing in a juice diet throughout the rest of your years.

Get Off on the Right Foot

Getting your body ready for a juicing diet is extremely crucial. Remember that you will be taking many things away from your body that it has grown accustomed to. Begin by slowly removing the junk food and poor eating habits at least two weeks prior to your juice diet. Begin by experimenting with different vegetable and fruit juices; you will be able to see which ones are the most pleasing to your taste buds. When you feel the need for junk food, start slowly by taking a juice drink in its place. As your start date approaches, begin removing more of the junk food and replacing it with a healthy juice concoction that you've grown to like.

If you have done it already, start drinking more water than any other beverage. This will begin the slow process of removing toxins from your system and preparing your colon with the needed lubricants that will be used during the detoxification process.

Begin taking a fiber supplement to keep your digestive system functioning in top form.   The quicker you get through the beginning stages of detoxification, the easier your juicing diet will be to endure.

Lastly, when you have finally reached your start date and are strictly juicing, stick with the juices that taste the most pleasant.   For the first few days, it would behoove you to mix in a wide variety of juices that you are unfamiliar with.   This will only fuel your level of quitting because, let's face it, the most healthy of juices are also the most unpleasant to drink.   Just drink the juice that will enable you to move forward.

With that being said, do not drink just fruit juice.   There are plenty of exciting tasting vegetable juices for you to choose from.   If you happen to find one that you seriously want to reap the benefits from, but the taste is awful to you, then mix a little of your favorite juice to give the drink a better taste.   Only mix in enough to make it taste agreeable to you.   Over juicing on fruits will leave your insulin levels high due to the sugar content of fruit and will reap havoc on your teeth because of the citric acid most fruits contain.   Above all, drink plenty of water during your entire juicing diet.   A recommended amount would be around a gallon of water a day or more.

You Need Variety

Once you have gotten over the hump of consuming only juice, you may find your diet a little boring.   This is another main reason why people quit juicing.   They simply become bored with the juice they are drinking and their urges for something different to taste becomes too overwhelming to ignore.   At the first sign of boredom, immediately begin experimenting with different fruit and vegetables. You can also try different juicing recipes.   There are recipes available that will blend a variety of fruits and vegetables together to give you a totally new taste sensation.   You will run out of time before you run out of different juicing recipes.   If you stick with this bit of advice, boredom will not be an issue for you while you're juicing.

Find a Juicing Partner

As with any diet or program, finding a partner to lean on during your times of weakness is immensely beneficial to your overall success. Even the most veteran of juicers find times of weakness and having someone to talk us through it is tremendously beneficial. You are not the only one that will need someone to talk to. Your partner will feel the same weaknesses that you may feel and will need to lean on you too. Sometimes, getting someone through a difficult time will not only help out the person seeking support, it will strengthen your dedication to your own program.

Cut Back on the Exercise

This can be a significant step toward your ultimate success. In regards to considering taking it slow, that doesn't mean to sit simply around. What this is meant to convey is that you will feel quite lethargic and weak at points of detoxification. During those times, and those times only, just allow yourself the rest you require.

At times of high energy, feel free to undertake your normal activities, even if those activities include exercising. The side-effect of juicing is that your body will begin to burn muscle instead of fat in order to maintain the protein levels it requires. There is much more energy burning protein in muscles than fat so, your body will seek out and use those areas first. Exercising during your energy bursts will effectively replace the loss muscle when you have your low-energy periods.

On the flip side, when you're feeling lethargic and weak, keep still and rest. The more you move during this time means the more muscle your body will begin to use in order to keep up with the demands for energy you've put on it. The reason you feel weak and lazy is that your body is using all the available energy for detoxification.

Once the detoxification period has passed, then that energy is built up, and you will feel an energy burst. Simply allow your body to work through those down times, and you'll feel better when you get to the other side.

Know When to Stop

Just as critical as preparing yourself for a juice diet, knowing when to stop juicing is just as crucial. If you continue juicing after one or more of these problems become more severe, the result could lead to organs shutting down, hospitalization, or in severe cases, death.

Understanding your body and the warning signs of serious distress could potentially save your life. However, keep in mind that you are detoxifying your body. You will most assuredly go through some of these side-effects as part of the detoxification process. Just know when these side-effects become more serious in nature.

Light headedness:

This side-effect is particularly common because of the lack of caloric intake you'll be receiving along with the detoxification of your body. When this becomes too severe, begin slowly by eating a small bowl of soup with no solids in it, something along the lines of tomato soup. If the condition becomes elevated to a point that you can't even stand-up for any length of time, seek medical attention.

Decreased Weight:

Naturally, this will happen due to the cleansing process along with the lower calorie consumption. Most of the initial weight loss will be in the form of water, so it will come off fairly quickly. You'll be hungry, but when your body goes through the stage of ketosis, then you might find yourself not hungry at all. If you're hunger feeling stays away for a long time, more than a week, and you keep losing weight, seek medical attention.   These are signs that you are in the process of starvation.

Low Blood Pressure:

Your blood pressure will go down due to the less stress that your body will be undergoing.   At times, your blood pressure may even elevate because of the toxins leaving your body.   A low blood pressure is a healthy sign to a healthy heart, but if it goes too low, it's also a sign that your heart may be in the process of shutting down. You'll know when your blood pressure becomes too low because you'll have a hard time even staying awake.   Monitor your blood pressure throughout your juicing diet.   If it goes too low and stays there, seek medical attention right away.

Hunger Pains:

You'll have these because your body will not be ingesting any solid foods.   Becoming accustomed to having solids in it, it inherently will growl and gurgle which will send hunger pains racing through your body.   Oftentimes, these pains will go away and only surface from time to time while juicing.

If your hunger pains send your pain level skyrocketing, and won't go away or go to your lower back, seek medical attention immediately.   There may be other issues going on inside your body that you know.

Loose Bowel Movement:

Another sign that the detoxification process is working, keep an eye on your bowel movements.   This could easily lead to dehydration.   If you continue having loose bowel movements long after all solids are removed from your system, if uncontrollable thirst persists, or any other signs of dehydration present itself, seek medical attention immediately.

Nausea:

As part of the detoxification process your body will be going through, occasional nausea may develop. Your body has become dependent on the toxins that are coursing through it, and when those are being removed, it can be compared to a smoker or drug user going through withdrawals. If your nausea persists well into the juice diet, other problems may be surfacing, and you should consult with your doctor or physician.

Kidney Ailments:

This side-effect can become quite serious if ignored. Your kidneys may feel the effects of detoxification, also. If consuming more water, cranberry juice, or other kidney specific juice drink doesn't help within a couple of days, seek medical attention. This could be a part of dehydration and your kidneys may be in the beginning stages of shutting down.

Arrhythmias:

Considering that your body will be undergoing a tremendous amount of stress, some heart arrhythmias may be normal. Persistent or exceeding painful ones need to be checked by a doctor. Do not think that they will simply ease or go away. Remember, it's your heart. Do not risk the waiting game with it.

As you can see, many side-effects are perfectly normal while some can be terribly serious if ignored. Always stay safe and don't be afraid to go just have it checked-out. When you do visit your doctor, be sure to let them know that you're performing a juice diet, how long you've been on it, what side-effects you've been feeling (all of them), and any other pertinent information about your health. If you are on a juice diet for diabetics, especially let them know this.

Who Can't Be on a Juice Diet?

While a juicing diet can be quite beneficial to your overall health, there are some individuals who must either modify the juice diet to fit a health concern, must wait to undergo a juice diet, or must not be on a juice diet at all. If you have one of the below health concerns, you are considered a "risk" to be on a juice diet. Please consult a doctor or physician to see if you can safely be on a juice diet, or need to modify a juice diet, to suit your personal health concerns.

Also, a juice diet can bring out an unknown health concern. A straightforward example of a health concern that is sometimes discovered is particular allergies to a certain food or food group. Consulting with your doctor or physician may make these unknown health concerns a known fact after basic tests are performed.

Individuals who are presently taking a prescription medicine. A juice diet may influence the drug you are prescribed in an unknown manner. Talking with your doctor or physician may bring to surface any unknown about the medicine.

Malnourished individuals do not need to partake in a juicing diet. The main side-effect is a welcomed one by many, losing weight. But if you are already malnourished and underweight, you do not need to lose any further weight.

Drug dependent people of people that are addicted to drugs must not participate in a juice diet. As with any drug, juicing will make these drugs act in a variety of ways that will be unhealthy to the body and may cause fatality.

Anemic people must not be on a juice diet without consulting their doctor or physician first. The blood system will undergo drastic changes during this time and may be particularly harmful to your body.

People that have undergone recent surgery, or are scheduled for a surgery must not be on a juice diet.   Your body is in a weak state during a juice diet and prior to, or after a surgery, your body must be in the healthiest and strongest possible state in order to heal itself. Juicing will not give your body the needed proteins for the healing process to begin.

Pregnant or nursing women must not be on a juicing diet.   Your body needs vital nutrients in order for the baby or fetus to be healthy and produce breast milk.   Without these vital nutrients, your baby may not develop correctly in the womb and your breast may not produce suitable milk, if it produces milk at all.

Individuals with any other serious medical condition such as diabetes, kidney, or liver illnesses must not undergo a juice diet without consultation with their doctor or physician first.   Your doctor or physician may have a specific diet or medicine that will coincide with the juice diet or tell you that you cannot do it at all.

If you have any of the above, please do not go on a juice diet blindly.   Talk about it with your doctor and weigh your options.   If they tell you not to go on one, please listen to them.   If you decide to undergo a juice diet without your doctor's approval, you may be risking your own life.   It's not worth it.

Exercising While Juicing

While it is recommended to not over-exert yourself while on a juicing diet, depending on the type of juicing diet you're on, you may be able to conduct your normal exercise routine.   Exercising while juicing is principally dependent upon the individual's requirements and exercise plan.   As with any questions about juicing for your personal needs, always consult with a doctor and let them know all the information about your juicing diet, and what kind of exercise routine you normally perform.

If you are juicing for pure health reasons, most "for health" juicing diets may not give you the necessary nutrients and proteins that are required for exercising. Juicing for health diets oftentimes decrease most everything within your body, so the toxins and pollutants will be flushed out. This will leave your body in a state of weakness for the time. However, discussing your exact juicing diet with your doctor may bring additional nutrient and protein values to light that you didn't know where available. They may even know of a different type of juicing diet that will be specifically designed for your body type and exercise requirements.

If you are juicing to lose weight, many juicing diets of this type will give you the necessary nutrients and proteins for you to be able to exercise. As with any diet for losing weight, exercise plays a critical component in the fat burning process. It is recommended to discuss with your doctor before going on any juice diet for weight loss and especially if you are planning on dieting while on the juice diet. Obvious health issues may need to be discussed prior to undergoing such a diet plan. Not so obvious reasons may surface that your doctor will be able to discuss with you.

Regardless of which type of juicing diet you will be taking part in, if you can exercise while on it, if the exercising leaves your body feeling downright exhausted and dehydrated, stop exercising immediately. If your doctor tells you that it's okay to move forward with your exercising routine, your body may be going through a serious detoxification process and is currently using that extra energy for the removal of toxins. Listen to your body and don't push it. Your body will let you know when you've had enough. If you go beyond your limits during this time, you may be doing more harm to your health than you're doing to improve it.

Juicing Recipes

There are many recipes for you to choose from regardless of which type of juicing diet you decide to undergo. Here, are a few basic recipes to get you started. It will show you just how recipes are set-up and measured. Some of these may get your taste buds going while others may bring a bit of a sour or, "not so good" taste to your mouth.

Fruit Recipes

Simple Apple Juice

3 Large Apples

Cut the stems off the apples and mix both tart and sweet tasting apples together for a fresh, refreshing "sweet and sour" apple juice. Keeping the peels on the apples will vastly increase the antioxidant, Flavonoid, level of the juice. The skin of fruits protects the fruit from sun exposure by acting like a container of sorts.

Simple Orange Juice

5 Large Oranges

Peel the oranges as you normally would. Grab as much of the white pith as you can so you can increase the antioxidant, Flavonoid, level of the juice. Do not juice the peel of the orange. The peel will make your juice go from a refreshing juice to an awful tasting juice.

The Best Lemonade

2 to 3 Large Lemons

½ Cup Purified Water
1 Medium Apple for Sweetness (Optional)

Peel the lemons and remove the stem from the apple, if you are adding one.   For limeade, simply substitute the apple with 1 lime.   Just add ice for a lovely, crisp drink on hot days.

Good Morning Blend

3 Kiwis
2 Cups Blueberries

Peel rind off kiwis and wash blueberries.   Place it all in your juicer and enjoy.   A great drink to kick off your day.   Kiwi fruit is loaded with Vitamin C, which keeps the immune system strong, to keep illness at bay and the skin tight to combat wrinkles.   Vitamin C is essential to the body producing collagen.   Collagen is the material that keeps skin cells together which produces a young and elastic skin appearance.

"Have a Berry Good Afternoon" Fruit Smoothie

2 Cups Strawberries
2 Cups Blueberries
1 ½ Cups Raspberries

Wash all berries thoroughly and juice.   A marvelous afternoon treat to refuel your body from the morning's activities.   Berries are a tremendous source of the antioxidant, anthocyanins.   Anthocyanins strengthen the arteries and protect them from oxidative damages. The antioxidant, ellagic acid, can also be found in berries and aid in cancer prevention.

Vegetable Recipes

"The Kicker"

3 Large Carrots
1 Beet
1/2" Fresh Ginger
1 Garlic Clove

Wash all vegetables and place in juicer. The "Kicker" juice recipe will get your taste buds going with a blend of delightful vegetables that, when eaten separately, may not be too pleasing to the palate. Blend them all together and you've got one magnificent tasting veggie juice drink!

"The Cleanser"

2 Large Celery Stalks
1 Handful of Kale
1 Handful of Spinach
1 Handful of Parsley
1 Ounce of Wheatgrass Juice

Wash all vegetables and place in juicer. This drink may not be too pleasing to your palate, but your body will thank you for it. Loaded with detoxifying nutrients, it will leave you body feel clean and toxin free within a matter of days.

"The Hydrator"

1 Large Celery Stalk
1 Medium Cucumber
1 Large Green Pepper
2 Handfuls of Spinach

Wash all vegetables and juice. The photonutrients that all of the green veggies contain will rehydrate your entire body within a short amount of time. Great drink if you're feeling thirsty.

"Just Like V8" Juice

2 Large Tomatoes
1 Medium Carrot
1 Large Celery Stalk
2 Leaves Lettuce
A Handful of Spinach
½ Handful of Parsley

Wash and juice all vegetables. If done in correct measurements, this juice will taste like store bought V8 Juice, only better. The nutrient level within this juice has not been altered or diminished during normal food processing. You'll have an appreciable tasting juice drink with all the benefits. Great morning starter.

"Sweet Juice"

3 Large Carrots
2 Medium Red Bell Peppers
2 Beets

Wash and juice all vegetables. This juice will taste exceptionally sweet; the sugar level is fairly low. Great for anyone that wants to be on an all vegetable juice diet, but still has a sweet tooth.

Both Fruit and Vegetable Recipes

"Body Rebuild"

1 Cup Spinach

1 Cucumber
2 Stalks Celery with Leaves still attached
3 Medium Carrots
½ Apple

Wash all vegetables and apple and juice together. Do not peel cucumber. Cucumber skin is loaded with nutrients, to rebuild red blood cells, and extremely healthy for skin. The apple addition gives the juice a neat pleasantly sweet taste.

"Cucumber and Apple Medley"

2 ½ Large Apples
1 Medium Cucumber
1" Ginger

Wash and combine all ingredients in juicer. Do not peel skins. Juice with skins on for additional nutrients that are trapped in the skins. Great juice for joint pain relief.

"The Crapple"

2 Medium Carrots
1 Large Red Apple
1" Ginger

Wash and juice all ingredients. Top the carrots and remove the stem from the apple, but don't peel anything. Another notable joint pain relief drink that is also renowned for your eyes!

"A Battery in a Glass"

2 Large Apples
1 Medium Cucumber
½ Peeled Lemon
½ Cup Kale

½ Cup Spinach
¼ Celery Bunch
¼ Fennel Bulb
1" Ginger
¼ Romaine Lettuce Head

Wash and juice all ingredients with skins on, except for the lemon. Great juice to recharge your energy level with pure, natural ingredients. Enjoy this juice for that mid-afternoon pick-me-up!

"Sweet Fruit and Veggie" Juice

1 Large Cucumber
1 Red Apple
1 Green Apple
¼ Cup Parsley
¼ Cup Mint
1 Celery Stalk
½" Ginger
½ Peeled Lemon

Wash and juice all ingredients.   Keep skin on all ingredients, except for lemon.   Exceptional juice that will satisfy any sweet-tooth!

Guide to Choosing the Best Juicing Equipment

When deciding which juicer to buy for your juicing diet, there are many questions that you'll need to ask.   Choosing the right juicer isn't as straightforward as "which brand to buy."   There are many different brands to choose from, and all of them have their own specific advantages and disadvantages.   The only basic differences between then are the "style" of juicer, the price, and ease of use.

What many individuals that are new to juicing don't always realize is that there isn't one particular juicer that will give you everything you want it to do. You'll have to "lose" something in order to "gain" something out of a juicer. This is why, you may see a few different juicers sitting on the bar at your local juice bar or at the kitchen of a friend's house. Each one will perform a different function in relation to the type of fruit or vegetable they are juicing. The three basic types of juicers are the centrifugal, the masticating, and the auger.

The centrifugal juicer relies on a single blade spinning at a high rotation per minute (RPM) and throws the cut fruit or vegetable against a spinning strainer. The strainer is where the juice is actually extracted from and fed into an awaiting spout that it comes out of.

The masticating juicer has a set of rotating blades that spin in opposite directions. The rotating blades simply cut that fruit or vegetable into extremely small pieces until all juice is extracted from the fibers. The juice is then poured directly from the blade section to a spout.

The last kind of juicer actually has two "sub-types" associated with it. It is the auger juicer and comes in a single-auger style or a double-auger style. These augers act like screws and pull the fruit or vegetable into it. The result is that the food is cut and pressed into a strainer and then to the awaiting spout.

However, like previously stated, each style has its pro's and con's about them. Leafy vegetables and small fruit berries won't be juiced exceptionally well in a centrifugal juicer while auger style juicers require more time to juice fruits and vegetables and are much harder to clean, but produces a higher yield and healthier juice. Centrifugal juicers aren't without their own benefits though. Masticating juicers offer a higher yield than others, but is harder to clean, more dangerous to clean, due to the exposed blades, and takes longer to produce the same volume of juice.

This is where all of the questions come into play. What kind of fruits and vegetables are you going to be juicing? How much juice will you be juicing all at once? Will you be storing the juice? How much time do you have in your schedule for juicing? Are you new to juicing? Does "foam" bother you when in a drink? By answering each of these questions, you'll be able to narrow down your choices on which juicer to purchase. Try to decide on one that will give you as much as you can without purchasing another juicer.

As mentioned already, no single juicer will give you all of what you want it to do. Concessions must be considered and made in order to find your "perfect" juicing equipment.

Centrifugal Juicer

If you happen to be looking for an easy, convenient, and cheap method for your initial juicing adventure, then the centrifugal juicer is the best way to go. They are fairly inexpensive, a variety of stores have them on the shelves; they're easy to use; produce a decent amount of juice within a short amount of time, and are easy to clean-up.

They're perfect for the beginner juicer that is just getting the hang of juice dieting. The one significant drawback it has is the juice tends to "go rancid" in a short amount of time. The process of spinning the food to release the juice puts air in the juice. Once air gets in it, the juice will almost immediately begin creating bacteria that will turn the juice a dark color.

Think of a cut apple slice. When you leave it for a short amount of time, it begins to turn brown in color. This is the same effect the juice has from a centrifugal juicer. Also, the air that is in the juice makes it appear foamy. If foam tends to bother you, then you'll find it hard to drink any juice from a centrifugal juicer.

On the positive side, the centrifugal juicer juices a sizeable amount of food in a short amount of time. This is due to the high RPM's it works at. If you're pressed for time, and need a glass of juice that you'll drink immediately, then the centrifugal juicer will do perfect for you. Another positive is that the centrifugal juicer is extremely easy to clean-up. A single-blade and basket-style strainer is essentially all it is, and they are fairly easy and quick to disassemble.

Masticating Juicers

Although these are an extremely early style of juicer, they can still be bought. The masticating juicer has several prominent qualities while having remarkably little downside. The opposing blades rotate at a low RPM and the motor is air cooled, so that means that you can juice with it for extended periods of time. The juice quality and quantity are high with this style, too.

One of the drawbacks is that, because the motor is air-cooled, the motor and blades tend to produce heat. This heat is then transferred to the juice in the juicer. When cleaning it, the blades are extraordinarily sharp, so you have to be extremely careful. Some masticating juicers aren't that easy to disassemble for clean-up, either. Foam is still an issue with it due to the spinning of the blades, which means that air is mixed with the juice, and we already know what air can do to juice.

Auger-Style Juicer

Probably the closest of all choices for the perfect juicer, that is, if you're a veteran juicer. It still takes a long time to juice foods, and some foods need to be pushed into the augers. If hard foods, such as carrots or any root vegetables, aren't actually pressed by hand into the augers, then they will simply bounce around on the top of it. If you are weak in your forearms or have wrist problems, this could drastically change your juicing regimen.

Leafy and small foods are juiced terrifically in it. While it still takes longer than the centrifugal juicer to produce juice, the auger-style juicer doesn't mix air into the juice which leaves the juice in a much healthier state. This is called drinking "living" juice because all of the vital nutrients are still in it. Being that the process actually "presses" the food into a strainer to acquire the juice, the amount of juice you'll receive is greater.

Clean-up is a significant pain and disassembly is a nightmare with the auger-style juicer. This is why it is only recommended for veteran juicers that know juicing equipment.

In summary, there is a variety of different juicing equipment for you to choose from. Think about, how you will use it and what will work best for you. Don't worry about which company made the juicer and certainly don't believe all the hype surrounding any ad about a juicer. Make the juicing equipment fit you instead of you fitting the juicing equipment. What may be beneficial for one person may not be advantageous for another.

Having the best or most expensive juicer money can buy is no good if you don't actually enjoy using it. If you find it hard or a hassle to even juice your fruits and vegetables, then you will never know the benefits of juicing. Buy juicing equipment that you'll actually use because it's not the equipment, but the juice that will make the difference in your life.

Juicing has been a longtime part of the human diet. We are turning to the "quick" meal instead of the "healthy" meal for our dietary needs. Our health has gone down drastically, and our bodies are struggling just to perform simple, everyday tasks because of the choices we make. There is hope for our bodies, and it can be found in juice.

Within these pages, you will discover a diet that our ancestors had the benefits of, and you will rediscover how our bodies were designed to work. Everything you need to know to prepare and conduct your own personally designed juicing program is in here. With a full history of juicing, who can juice, what to juice, what ailments it helps, how to lose weight with juice and fabulous juicing recipes, your juicing program will be an enjoyable success—the type of success that will last you a lifetime. Change your life with juicing!

101 Juice Diet Recipes

Aromatic Juice Drink

This juice is loaded with vitamins and minerals that are good for the heart; help reduce blood cholesterol, and lower blood pressure. Rich in vitamin C and B-complex that helps the body develop immune resistance, improve the intestinal motility and has anti-inflammatory, painkiller, nerve soothing, anti-pyretic as well as anti-bacterial properties. This is a refreshing and aromatic juice drink.

1 cucumber
1 mango
2 stalk fennel with leaves
1 sprigs of mint
1/2 inch piece of ginger

Push all through the juicer. Note: mint leaves can be rolled up into a ball to create volume when pushing through the juice extractor. Stir and enjoy!

Celery Cucumber Cooler
Celery and cucumber are low-calorie vegetables but rich sources of dietary fiber, an ideal combination for weight loss. This is a refreshing mix of fruits and vegetables which are all rich in vitamins and anti-oxidants. This cooler can help reduce inflammation and give protection against cancer.

3 stalk celery
½ medium cucumber, peeled
2 apple, sliced
5 medium carrots, greens removed
1 lemon, sliced

Combine all ingredients together in the juicer, stir and serve.

Healing Juice

If you are suffering from high blood pressure, having blurry vision and heart problems, this is a healing juice for you. Vegetables are a rich source of vitamins and anti-oxidants to cure various health problems.

4-5 medium carrots
100g fresh spinach
100g leaf parsley
4-5 sticks of celery

Combine all ingredients together in the juicer. Stir and serve.

Mediterranean Juice

This is a recommended drink for those suffering from anemia since these vegetables are a rich source of iron along with other vitamins and minerals.

100g parsley
1-2 red pepper
1-2 cups broccoli florets
4 medium carrots

Put ingredients through juicer in the same order as the list. Add flavor in the mix with lemon and orange juice if desired. Stir and serve.

The Big C Fighter

This combination of fruits and vegetables are rich in phytochemicals known to fight carcinogens which may cause cancer. A good source of vitamins, minerals and dietary fiber as well which helps to improve general health.

2 stalks broccoli
½ head of cabbage
½ head of cauliflower
50g spinach
½ lime
3 peaches

Core the peaches and cut a lime in half. Prepare the cabbage and cauliflower. Juice the broccoli, cabbage, cauliflower, spinach, lime and peaches together and serve.

Very Berry Power

Berries contain phytochemicals and flavonoids that may reduce the risk of getting cancer. Blackberries and blueberries specifically are rich in minerals that may prevent bladder infections. This juice mix is a low-calorie source of vitamins and anti-oxidants.

1 cup blackberries
2 cups blueberries
2 apples, cored and sliced

Process the fruits in a juicer and serve.

Berry Akai Delight

The acai berry is loaded with phytochemicals known to reduce the risk of cancer, cardiovascular illness and lessen the severity of common ailments such as colds and flu.

½ cup acai berries
½ lemon
½ papaya (peeled)

1 ½ tablespoon honey

Put them all in a juicer and enjoy!

Super Anti-oxidant

Raspberry is a super fruit packed with anti-oxidants, vitamins C, minerals and fibers. The combination of spinach, peach, lime and cucumber make this concoction a super anti-oxidant.

1 cup raspberry
1 ½ cup spinach
1 peach
½ lime
1/2 cucumber

Wash all the ingredients. Run them through a juicer. Take the expelled pulp and run it back through the juicer a second time to extract all liquid. Serve and drink.

Super Colon Cleanser

This juice is loaded with phytochemicals and nutrients as well as dietary fibers that are good for colon and gallbladder cleansing.

2 apples
½ medium carrots
4 slices of medium cucumber
2 stalks of celery
½ tbsp of honey

Mix the apple, celery, carrot, cucumber, lemon juice and honey in your juicer. Puree into a shake.

Drink immediately before it oxidizes.

Cholesterol Fighter

This nutritious drink is low in cholesterol but rich in anti-oxidants, vitamins, minerals and dietary fiber which helps control blood cholesterol levels, prevents constipation, protects body from free radicals mediated injury and from cancers.

5 carrots
7 stalks celery with leaves
8 stems parsley with leaves
3 garlic cloves

Juice all the ingredients together and you're done. Stir and serve.

Cleansing Veggie Combi

Rich in vitamins and minerals, vegetables are also a good source of dietary fiber which is a natural body cleanser. This combination of vegetables is ideal for a weight loss regimen since they are all low in calories.

2 cups kale leaves
2 stalks celery
1cup beets
1 turnip
½ cup spinach
½ head bokchoy
2 cups parsley
2 garlic cloves

Juice all ingredients in a juicer until smooth. Drink up and enjoy!

Liver Cleansing Juice Drink

Over exposure to toxins may over-stress the liver and affect the other organs resulting to common symptoms such as headaches, muscle pain, fatigue, poor coordination, nerve problems, skin irritations and emotional imbalances. This juice can help cleanse the liver from harmful toxins. Loaded with anti-oxidant compounds, it can also help boost immune system and protect the body against cancer.

2 cups grape
5 stalks chard
1 grapefruit
½ lime

Process all ingredients in a juicer. Stir and enjoy!

Fiery Fruity Drink

Chili peppers have amazingly high levels of vitamins and minerals. They specifically contain capsaicin which has anti-bacterial, anti-carcinogenic, analgesic and anti-diabetic properties. They also help reduce the cholesterol levels in the blood.

2 whole green peppers
2 ¼ tbsps. of honey
½ lime
1 apple

Clean the chili peppers and remove the seeds. Peel the lime and wash the apple. Mix the apple, chili peppers and lime in the juicer. Then add the honey into the finished juice until it fully dissolves. Stir and drink.

Everyday Energizer

Low in calories but a good source of energy boosting vitamins, this juice drink is recommended to prevent cancer and booster immunity. Also high in fiber, including the soluble type that lowers elevated blood cholesterol levels.

4 carrots
5 stalks celery
1 cup of parsley
1 cup squash, zucchini

1 small beet chopped
½ inch ginger
½ lemons peeled

Push all ingredients through the juicer and drink up!

Juice Detox

This delicious fruit mix is loaded with vitamins and minerals to cleanse the body and remove toxins and free radicals.

2 cups grapes
2-3 cups strawberries
3 apricots
3 sprigs fresh mint

Combine all ingredients together in the juicer.   Stir and serve.

Skin Cleanser

If you are suffering from skin break-outs, this juice mix can help clear your skin. Cucumber has a cooling and hydrating effect on the skin and combined with the other vegetables which are rich in vitamins and anti-oxidants, your skin will surely benefit from this mix.

1 ½ cucumber with skin
1 cup fresh parsley
½ cup chopped alfalfa sprouts
4 sprigs fresh mint

Combine all ingredients together in the juicer.   Stir and serve.

Sweet and Tangy Drink

This juice recipe combines the taste of earthy vegetables and sweetness of fruits with tangy kale. Rich in anti-oxidants and high in fiber, this is a nutrient-packed drink for the health conscious.

8 medium carrots

2 cups kale leaves
1½ cup turnip
1½ cup parsnip
7 stalks celery
1 rutabaga
¼ head red cabbage.
6 radishes
1 apple
1 cup cranberry

Process the ingredients one by one in a juicer. Combine and enjoy!

The Milk Alternative

Broccoli and kale are an excellent source of calcium and Vitamin K needed for bone health. Along with carrots and apple, this mix is an excellent source of anti-oxidants, vitamins and dietary fiber. As a milk alternative, this is even better than milk.

1 cup broccoli florets
2-3 kale leaves
3-4 medium-sized carrots
Half slice of an apple

Wash carrots thoroughly and remove tops. Put all ingredients together in the juicer, stir and chill.

Fruity Berry

Berries are loaded with antioxidants that help to prevent cancer. They are also loaded with vitamins and minerals to help strengthen arteries and protect them from oxidative damage.
3 cups of strawberries
3 cups of blueberries
1½ cup of choke berry
Wash thoroughly and juice. Drink and enjoy!

Carrot and Ginger Cleanser

Carrots are a good source of beta-carotene, an anti-oxidant and immune booster. This juice blend is rich in dietary fiber, a natural internal body cleanser.

3 cups carrots
½ inch of fresh ginger root
1 orange

Peel the ginger root and carrot before placing them in the juicer. Stir the juice. Serve cold with slices of orange and drink!

Alkaline Juice

Over-acidity in the body tissues can cause arthritic and rheumatic diseases. Symptoms of over-acidity include insomnia, water retention, migraines, and fatigue. Eating alkalizing fruits and vegetables can effectively relieve these symptoms.

1 cucumber peeled
3 stalks of celery
1 ½ Large handfuls of turnip greens
3 cloves of garlic peeled
½ lemon peeled

Push all through the juicer. Juice the greens by pushing them down with the cucumber or celery.

Banana Almonds Smoothie

This is a delicious energy-booster drink rich in dietary fiber, vitamins, and minerals and packed with numerous health promoting phytochemicals that ensure protection against diseases and cancers.

1cup plum
2 small banana
1 ½ cup fresh rhubarb
1 ½ tsp. of honey

Process all ingredients in a juicer until smooth. Drink and enjoy!

Blood Pressure Regulator

This is a recipe loaded with anti-oxidants, vitamin C and dietary fiber. This juice can help regulate blood pressure and lower cholesterol as well.

4-5 stalks fresh bokchoy
4-5 stalks of celery
1 ½   cucumber
2 cups fresh spinach leaves
2 ½   apples

Wash vegetables and fruit. Cut all except spinach into smaller pieces to fit into juicer. Put all through juicer. Spinach leaves may be wrapped around the veggies or rolled up to make them easier to juice. Stir and serve.

Bone Strengthener Detox

This is a low calorie juice drink which can help strengthen the bones, and loaded with anti-oxidants to help fight certain kinds of cancer as well. Great for body detox.

1 ½ heads cauliflower
2 cups butternut squash cut into desired size
1/2 lemon
1 apple
2 cups spinach
3 stalks celery with tops
¼ cup romaine lettuce
1 bulb fennel
½ cube ginger
2 cloves garlic

Wash all veggies and run them through the juicer. Run the pulp back through the juicer a second time. Serve and enjoy.

Applelicious Veggie Drink

Apples are low in calories but contain good quantities
of vitamin-C and beta-carotene which is a powerful natural antioxidant
and helps the body develop resistance against infectious diseases.
Vegetables are also loaded with antioxidants that protect the body from
oxidant stress and cancers, as well as help boost the immune system.

2 ripe apples
½ cup spinach
1 cup parsley
3 stalks celery
7 stalks napa cabbage

Wash the stuff, cut into small sections if needed. Juice the apples and
set aside. Juice all the remaining ingredients. Add the apples, stir and
enjoy.

Pumpkin Power Drink

Pumpkin, by itself, is a storehouse of anti-oxidant vitamins such as A,
C and E that helps the body develops resistance against infectious
agents and protects it against lung and oral cavity cancers. Added with
apple and carrots, this juice combination is a powerhouse of
anti-oxidants which also gives protection against damage from free
radicals that causes premature ageing.

3 cups pumpkin chunks
2 loquat
3 carrots
1 inch piece ginger
cinnamon
small amount of nutmeg

Cut the pumpkin in half and scoop out the seeds. Cut into 1 1/2 inch chunks and remove skin with a vegetable peeler. Wash apple and carrots and cut into pieces that will fit into your juicer. Put the first four ingredients through your juicer. Pour the juice into a glass and sprinkle with cinnamon and nutmeg. Add ice if desired. Makes approximately 12 oz.

Green Delight

This juice blend is a good source of anti-oxidants and dietary fiber for protection against certain types of cancer. Drinking this juice regularly helps prevent osteoporosis, relieve constipation and helps the body develop resistance against infectious diseases.

1 apple
2 cucumbers
½ green cabbage
2 cups spinach

Wash fruits and vegetables. Cut to the size that will fit in your juicer. Push the raw foods through the juicer machine. Add ice and enjoy. Makes approximately10 oz of juice.

The Colors of Summer

The combination of cantaloupe, apple and pineapple makes for a low-calorie drink loaded with anti-oxidant vitamins A and C. These are essential for vision, immunity, healthy mucus membranes and skin. Consumption of natural fruits rich in vitamin-A is known to protect from lung and oral cavity cancers. Rich in electrolytes and water content, this is an ideal nutritious drink to beat the summer thirst.

½ medium cantaloupe
2 medium apples
½ cup pineapple

Juice ingredients in a juicer until smooth. Drink and enjoy!

Three C's Plus One Juice Drink

This juice is low in calories and rich in vitamins, minerals and anti-oxidants that boost immune system. Drinking this mix can help lower homocysteine levels in the blood, high levels of which can result in the development of coronary heart disease, stroke and peripheral vascular diseases. The vitamin K specifically found in celery also help strengthens bones.

2 carrots
½ cup chard
3 sticks celery
2 cucumbers

Wash the stuff, cut into small sections if needed. Juice everything together until desired consistency. Stir and enjoy.

Green Cocktail

This juice blend is a storehouse of phytonutrients that promote good health and disease prevention properties. Loaded with vitamins A, B-complex, E and K as well as essential minerals to protect the skin from premature ageing and boost the immune system, this green cocktail is ideal for the health-conscious.

2 kale leaves
2 cups spinach
½ peach
½ fresh avocado
½ tbsp flax seed
2 cups green grapes

Process all ingredients in a juicer until smooth. Drink and enjoy!

Spicy Veggie Drink

This juice blend contains no cholesterol; but rich in anti-oxidants, vitamins, minerals, dietary fiber and other healthful substances which helps control blood cholesterol levels, prevents constipation, and protects the body against certain cancers.

1 bunch parsley
6 turnips
4 tomatoes
2 red bell peppers
2 onions
1 clove garlic

Wash and Combine all ingredients together in the juicer. Stir, enjoy and relax.

Fresh Vital Green Drink

Kale leaves contains more iron and calcium than most vegetable. Its high vitamin C- content enhances the body to absorb these minerals. This juice blend is also an excellent low-calorie source of lycopene, and anti-oxidant vitamins, minerals as well as dietary fiber that helps to control blood cholesterol levels, and helps fight the cancer-causing chemicals in our body.

3 cups kale leaf
3 cups collard leaf
3 cups parsley
½ green pepper
2 green tomatoes
1 floret broccoli

Wash then combine all ingredients together in the juicer. Stir and enjoy.

Armor Shield Drink

This juice combination is good source of dietary fiber, beta carotene, folate, vitamin A & C , calcium, potassium and iron that may protect against some intestinal upsets and may help prevent some urinary tract infections, prevent night blindness, ease arthritis pain and help reduce the risk of certain cancers. Try this juice combination in your fasting diet today.

1 cup blueberries
5 medium carrots
2 medium cucumbers
5 celery stalks
2cups beet
1 cup pineapple

Wash all the ingredients, peel the carrots and cucumbers. Combine all ingredients together in the juicer. Stir and serve.

Orangey Avocado Drink

This juice rich in numerous anti-oxidant polyphenolic flavonoids and contains essential fatty acids which are good for your heart and help reduce bad cholesterol. In addition to this, the avocado supplies you with a large quantity of fibers which are good for your digestion. Also, the orange and melon contains a high amount of vitamin C, which help strengthen the immune system.

1 avocado
1 melon
1 orange
4 stalks of fresh cilantro

Combine all ingredients in a juicer. Process and mix well. Add ice cubes, serve cold and enjoy.

Popeye Juice

This vegetable juice combination contains health-promoting

phytochemicals that helps protect the body against certain kinds of cancer. It is a very excellent source of vitamin A, C, K, calcium, iron, potassium, and anti-oxidants which are important as intracellular electrolyte, strengthening bone formation, immune system booster, blood pressure reducer and essential for red blood cell formation.

2 cups spinach

2 stalks kale

2 fennel bulbs

2 cups parsley

1 cucumber

1 one-inch cube of ginger

Wash all ingredients. Run them through a juicer. Any pulp should be run through the juicer a second time to extract all juice from the vegetables. Serve and drink.

Yummy Green Drink

Spinach is one of the vegetable recommended in cholesterol control and weight reduction. This vegetable and fruit juice combination is a very rich source of heart healthy electrolytes, antioxidant, vitamins and minerals that gives the body energy and immunity resistance against infectious diseases.

1 cup spinach
2 cups kale leaves
1 orange
2 banana
1 kiwi

Wash all ingredients thoroughly. Put all ingredients together in the juicer, stir and drink.

Heart-Friendly Juice

This delicious and refreshing juice drink is full of anti-oxidants which keep the bad cholesterol away, as well as buffer the effects of free radical damage to the cells caused by oxidation. Pomegranate seeds keep blood platelets from sticking together and forming dangerous blood clots and also increase oxygen levels to the heart. Mango is a very rich source of potassium that helps control heart rate and blood pressure.

2 pomegranates
½ mango
1 stalk mint

Peel the pomegranate and remove the seeds. Peel the mango, and put both mango and pomegranate in the juice press. Pour the juice in a large glass and add the mint and pomegranate seeds on top. Drink and enjoy.

Tropical Juice Drink

The papain in papaya, bromelain in pineapple, pectin in orange, astringent properties of guava and the polyphenolic anti-oxidant compounds in mango combine to make this the ultimate juice drink. Rich in essential vitamins and minerals as well as anti-oxidant compounds and dietary fiber, this juice is good for the heart and digestion, has anti-ageing properties, immune booster and anti-cancer, all in one.

2 mangoes
1 large orange
½ pineapple
½ big papaya
1 big guava

Combine all ingredients in the juicer. Stir and enjoy this delicious juice drink.

Berry Guava Mix

Berries contain phytochemicals and flavonoids that may help to prevent some forms of cancer. They are low in calories but rich in vitamins A and C. Guava is also rich in vitamin C as well as dietary fiber to help cleanse the colon.

1 ½ cup strawberry
1 ½ cup raspberries
1 ½ cup blackberries
½ big guava

Process ingredients in the juicer, drink and enjoy!

Asian Flavor Drink

This fruit combination is rich in anti-oxidant vitamins A, C and E, as well as flavonoids such as pectin, a soluble fiber that helps lower cholesterol and blood pressure.

2 pcs kumquat
1 pc tangerine
3 pcs pears
3 pcs apples

Wash all ingredients and run them through the juicer.   Stir, serve and enjoy this flavorful drink.

Chlorophyll Juice

Consuming chlorophyll from this juice is a highly effective way to alkalize the blood and energize the body. This juice is a great source of vitamins A, B, C, E, potassium, lutein and carotene which are highly effective in eliminating free radicals and prevent cancer of the lung and prostate. This juice combination has the ability to cleanse the blood, organs and gastrointestinal tract as well as help prevent blindness and lower blood cholesterol levels.

2 cups spinach
1 bunch wheat grass
6 carrots

1 stalk celery

Wash all ingredients and run them through the juicer. Run the pulp back through the juicer a second time. Drink and enjoy.

Tangy Berry Drink

This juice combination is loaded with vitamin C and bioflavonoids that help strengthen immune resistance, lower blood cholesterol and protect against cancer. Add this juice recipe in your diet fasting.

2 tangerines
1 cup raspberry
½ lemon
1 inch ginger

Wash all ingredients and run them through the juicer.   Stir, serve and enjoy.

Carroty Green Drink

Juice fasting does no harm and may at the same time confer major health benefits against two leading killers, cancer and heart disease. This juice blend are excellent source of beta carotene, dietary fiber, calcium, iron, potassium, vitamin A and C that help prevent night blindness, protect against cell damage by free radicals, reduce blood sugar levels in diabetics and help heal peptic ulcers.

6 medium carrots
1 bunch watercress
3 cups parsley
1 cup green cabbage

Wash all the ingredients thoroughly. Scrub the carrots and push them through the machine with the watercress leaves, parsley and its stalks and the cabbage. Drink immediately.

Spicy Fiber Drink

This nutritious juice for the weight-conscious is an excellent source of beta carotene and vitamins A, C and E, folate, calcium, and potassium as well as dietary fiber. This juice blend helps alleviate viral infections by boosting immunity. It also helps remove harmful free radicals from the body and protects it from certain kinds of cancer.

2 cups kale
3 apples
3 horseradish
½ lemon
1 stalk celery
½ inch ginger

Wash all ingredients and run them through the juicer.   Stir, serve and enjoy.

Refreshing Fruit Drink

An excellent source of vitamin A, C, beta carotene, folate, thiamine and potassium a nutrient essential for healthy hair, skin, eyes, bones, and mucous membranes, this refreshing juice has a menthol taste and a cooling sensation that helps reduce blood cholesterol and blood pressure level.

1 orange
3 carrots
½ papaya
3 apples
1 guava
½ cup peppermint

Wash all ingredients and run them through the juicer.   Stir, serve and enjoy.

Veggie Squeeze

This juice blend is an excellent source of antioxidant vitamins A and C as well as potassium that help prevents infections in the body and essential to the diet because they protect against cancer. Try this juice in your fasting diet for effective result.

5 carrots
2 cucumbers
3 stalks celery
2 asparagus
2 zucchinis

Wash all ingredients and combine together in the juicer. Stir and enjoy.

Sunshiny Drink

This juice combination is high in vitamin C and provides a good amount of pectin, a soluble dietary fiber that helps control blood cholesterol levels and boosts the immune system against diseases.

½ orange
2 grapefruit
¼ medium papaya
1 inch ginger

Wash all ingredients and run them through the juicer.   Stir, serve and enjoy.

Garden Delight

Collard greens are excellent source of vitamin-A and flavonoids that help improves healthy mucous membranes and skin, also essential for vision. This vegetable juice contains excellent amount of beta carotene, lycopene, folate, vitamin C, calcium, iron, potassium and antioxidants to prevent cancer-causing cell damage, control heart rate, reduce blood pressure, essential for body metabolism and blood cell formation.

4 stalks collard greens
2 cups romaine lettuce leaves
2 skinny carrots
1 cup cauliflower
1 large eggplant
2 stalks celery
3 small peppers
1 medium tomato

Add fresh ground black pepper to taste. Wash all ingredients and run them through the juicer. Stir, serve and enjoy.

Salad Drink

This juice blend is loaded with dietary fiber and vitamins A and C, folate, potassium and lycopene which helps increase bulk of the food by absorbing water throughout the digestive system and helps in easing constipation, treat gout, high blood pressure and protect against some cancers.

1 bunch coriander leaves
4 medium tomatoes
4 stalks celery
1 onion
3 green peppers

Wash all ingredients thoroughly. Put together in the juicer, stir and drink.

Rainbow Drink

This juice is a storehouse of phytonutrients that have health promotional and disease prevention properties. Loaded with vitamins A, B-complex, C, E, K, pyridoxine, carotenes, omega-fatty acids, riboflavin, and thiamine, this fruit blend helps to protect the body from harmful free radicals and boost the immune system, as well as being anti-inflammatory, anti-ulcer, and anti-cancer.

2 cups kale
2 cups spinach
2 cups lychee
½ fresh avocado
1 cup grapes
2 tbsp hemp seeds

Process all ingredients in a juicer until smooth. Drink and enjoy!

Flavonoid Drink

This juice blend is rich in fiber and flavonoids that helps lower body cholesterol level and improves blood flow. This is also an excellent source of anti-oxidant vitamins A, C and E as well as B-complex and beta carotene that boosts the immune system and protects the body against harmful free radicals.

2 kiwi fruits
2 star fruits
1 medium eggplant
1 medium cucumber

Wash all ingredients and run them through the juicer. Stir, serve and enjoy.

Juicy Greens

Celery, chard and kale are good sources of potassium, folate, calcium, omega-3 fatty acids and bioflavonoids that help protect against certain cancers, retain the elasticity of the arteries, as well as help improve the digestive system and lower cholesterol levels.

3 stalks celery
1 cup green Swiss chard leaf
5 kale leaves
½ pomelo
1 apple
¼ inch ginger

Push all ingredients through the juicer.   Juice the greens by pushing them down with fruits. Stir and enjoy.

Leafy Delight

This juice combination is a low-calorie source of dietary fiber that helps reduce weight while preventing constipation and colon-rectal cancer risks; decrease bad cholesterol levels and regulates blood sugar levels. This juice mix is full of antioxidant vitamins vitamin A, C, K and B-complex to protect the body against cancer, promote healthy mucus membranes and bone development as well as help the body develop resistance against infectious agents.

1 bunch asparagus
1 handful collard greens
2 stalks celery
1 carrot
1 apple

Wash all ingredients and run them through the juicer. Run the pulp back through the juicer a second time. Serve and enjoy.

Grapefruit Power Juice

Grapefruit contains salicylic acid that helps break down the body's inorganic calcium, which builds up in the cartilage of joints and may lead to arthritis. Sweet potatoes are high in vitamin B6 which helps prevent degenerative diseases including heart attacks. Peaches are rich in dietary fiber and potassium which acts as a kidney cleanser.   All three contain anti-oxidant vitamins and minerals which boost the immune system and fight harmful free radicals.

3 grapefruits
2 sweet potatoes
2 peaches

Process the ingredients in a juicer and serve.

Starry Starry Mix

This vegetable and fruit juice combination contains health-promoting phytochemicals that helps protect the body against certain kinds of diseases, especially the antioxidants and bioflavonoids that help block cancer causing substances. This juice is rich in ascorbic acid and bromelain, which is important to keep bones, teeth, mucous membranes, skin and immune system healthy. It also helps to reduce digestive upsets and reduce inflammation. Get your juicer now! Be healthy, be happy.

3 cups spinach
1 ½ star fruit
½ cup pineapples
3 medium cucumbers peeled

Wash all the ingredients. Run them through a juicer. Take the expelled pulp and run it back through the juicer a second time to extract all liquid. Stir and enjoy!

Sweet Melon Mint

This juice combination is a rich source of anti-oxidants such as vitamin C, beta-carotene and lutein which acts as protective scavengers against harmful free radicals that play a role in aging and various disease processes, and potassium which helps reduce blood pressure and heart rates by countering the effects of sodium.

½ honeydew melon
2 medium cucumbers
1 cup mint leaves
1 cup pineapple
3 medium eggplant peeled

Wash then combine all ingredients together in the juicer. Stir and enjoy.

Raisin Alert Mix

This juice combination is ideal for those suffering from high blood pressure, constipation problems, stress, obesity and a lot more. It helps to flush toxins inside the body; helps enhance the immune system and provide essential nutrients and anti-oxidants.

5 apples
3 carrots
½ cup raisins
2 tbsp honey

Wash all the ingredients thoroughly. Scrub the carrots and push them all through the machine. Drink immediately and relax.

Sweet Savory Juice

This juice combination is an excellent source of beta carotene, lycopene, vitamin A, C and potassium, which helps lower blood cholesterol levels and prevent certain cancer.

3 pcs large bell pepper
7 carrots
2 medium tomatoes
1 tbsp honey

Wash all ingredients except honey and run them through the juicer. Add honey and stir. Serve and enjoy.

Spare of Asparagus

This juice combination has the highest nutritional value especially for those people suffering from insomnia, irritable bowel syndrome, and blurred vision. This juice blend is also rich in potassium, copper and iron which are important components of cell and body fluids that helps control heart rate, blood pressure, cellular respiration and red blood cell formation.

5 asparagus
2 medium carrots
1 lemon
2 tomato
1 tbsp honey
Juice them all and serve!

Sweet Humid Drink

This juice blend is rich in dietary fiber that helps to protect the colon and mucous membrane, helps control heart rate and lower blood pressure. It is an excellent source of vitamins A and C, as well as potassium and beta carotene that help lower blood cholesterol levels, protect against cancer and prevent blindness.

2 cups ripe jackfruit bulbs
3 medium carrots
5 cups spinach
3 stalks celery
2 lemons
½ inch ginger

Wash all ingredients and run them through the juicer.   Stir and Enjoy!!

Peach Berry Cocktail

This juice combination provides some vitamin C, iron, potassium, beta carotene, folate and thiamine. It is high in fiber especially pectin, a soluble fiber that is instrumental in lowering high blood cholesterol.

3 peaches
2 orange
1cup blueberries
1 cup cherries

Push fruits through the juicer. Stir, serve and enjoy!

Disease Fighting Juice

This juice blend helps fight heart diseases, diabetes, constipation, cancer, arthritis and high blood pressure. It is rich in antioxidants, omega-3 essential fatty acids, vitamins A, C and K and other essential nutrients.

2 small banana
1 cup spinach
½ tbsp ground flaxseed
½ tbsp chia seeds
1 apple

Put in the juicer. Process and serve.

Sweet Freshener Juice Drink

Spinach is a rich source of vitamin A and lutein which keeps the eyes and mucous membranes. This juice is an abundant with beta carotene, vitamins A, C, E, K,folate, potassium and lycopene that help reduce the risk of macular degeneration, reduce inflammation and protect against cancer. Try this juice with its sweet and menthol taste which is good to relieve, asthma, fatigue and stress.

1 cup spinach
1 medium carrots
1 cup parsley
2 stalks celery
3 medium bell peppers
3 medium tomatoes
½ cup mint leaves
1 tbsp honey

Push all through juicer. Note: mint leaves can be rolled up into a ball to create volume when pushing through the juice extractor. Makes 12 oz of juice. Stir and enjoy!

Jalapeño Madness

Jalapeno pepper has a chemical compound called capsaicin which helps lower blood cholesterol, promotes weight loss and fights against some types of colon and stomach cancers.

2 jalapeno peppers
2 large green peppers
1 cup cilantro
2 green onions
3 large tomatoes
½ avocado

Wash all the ingredients. Run them through a juicer. Take the expelled pulp and run it back through the juicer a second time to extract all liquid. Drink and enjoy!

Green Vapors

The combination of spinach, lettuce, celery, carrots, cucumbers and a squeeze of lime is effective in body cleansing. Juice is better chilled as possible in the morning before living for work. Keep it cool to help minimize oxidation.

2 cups spinach
2 cups romaine lettuce
2 stalks celery
5 medium carrots
3 medium cucumbers
½ lime

Wash all the ingredients. Run them through a juicer. Take the expelled pulp and run it back through the juicer a second time to extract all liquid. Makes approximately 16 oz of juice. Stir and enjoy!

Body Toxin Cleanser

Dietary cholesterol is the type consumed in foods specifically animal products and junk foods. The body does not need this cholesterol; it can cause certain diseases. To wash out this type of toxin inside the body, try this juice combination. It is recommended as an effective body toxin cleanser.

1 medium apple
2 cups spinach
2 cups parsley
2 large carrots
1 cup celery leaves
1 medium beet root with green tops

Wash all the ingredients. Run them through a juicer. Take the expelled pulp and run it back through the juicer a second time to extract all liquid. Stir the juice and serve immediately for the greatest nutritional benefits.

Pea and Basil Juice

Besides being high in protein, fresh green peas are good sources of pectin and other soluble fiber, which help control blood cholesterol levels. This juice mix is full of digestion friendly fiber to help prevent cardiovascular disease and constipation.   It also contains many polyphenolic flavonoids known to have anti-inflammatory and anti-bacterial properties as well as high amount of iron which is very important in the production of healthy red blood cells.

1 cup sweet peas
3 stalks celery with leaves
1 tomato
½ garlic clove
5 cups basil leaves

Rinse the vegetables first and then put the peas, celery leaves and tomatoes into the juicer. Squeeze garlic with basil in a different container. Pour the juice into a glass, and mix in the garlic-basil. Stir and serve.

Pepper Bell

Fresh red and green peppers are rich source of vitamin C which is a potent water soluble antioxidant. It is required for the collagen synthesis in the body in maintaining the integrity of blood vessels, skin, organs, and bones. This juice is loaded with vitamins, minerals and antioxidants. This juice is good source of dietary fiber that helps reduce constipation, promote weight loss, helps control heart rate and blood pressure.

1green peppers
1 red pepper
2celery stalks
1cucumber
2 cups lettuce leaves

Wash thoroughly and combine all ingredients in the juicer. Stir and serve.

Fruit grass Combi

More than ever, people are realizing that what they eat does make a difference, not only in the way they look and feel but also in the length and quality of their lives. To obtain a healthy body, follow a healthy and balance diet. Try this juice combination for an effective body detoxification.

1 cup grapes
½ cup pineapple
½ cup wheat grass

Juice all the ingredients together and you're done. Stir and serve.

Orange Wheat

Try this juice with wheatgrass combination to help the body fight against common diseases and certain kinds of cancer. This combination is rich in antioxidant vitamins A, C and E which are important for immune function to ward off infection and assist in bonding cells and strengthening the blood vessel walls.

2 bunch wheatgrass
1 inch piece fresh ginger
5 pieces oranges

Wash all the ingredients. Run them through a juicer. Take the expelled pulp and run it back through the juicer a second time to extract all liquid. Stir juice and serve immediately for the greatest nutritional benefit.

Tomato Desire

This juice blend is an excellent low calorie source of vitamins A, C, potassium and lycopene. It can help lower the risk of prostate cancer in men and reduce inflammation. It also helps lower blood pressure and cholesterol levels.

3 ripe tomatoes
2 green peppers
2 stalks celery
2 apples
2 onions

Wash all ingredients and run them through the juicer. Run the pulp back through the juicer a second time. Serve and enjoy.

Walnut Harmony

Research has found consumption of small amounts of walnuts is linked to decreased risk of heart disease, certain kinds of cancer, gallstones, type 2 diabetes and other health problems.   This juice combination is rich in anti-oxidants which protect the body against the damaging effects of free radicals and other food chemicals.

4 apples
2 stalks celery with leaves
1 cup grapes
1 cup walnuts

Wash all ingredients thoroughly. Put all ingredients together in the juicer, stir and drink.

Alpha Mix

Juice fasting is highly recommended to relieve symptoms, maintain good health and promote healing, not to replace the medicines and surgery that doctors use to treat illness but to help them prevent the risk of the disease and help the immune system to fight illnesses. This juice blend is a storehouse of phytonutrients that promote good health and disease prevention properties.

2 medium sweet potatoes peeled
2 orange
2 red capsicum
2 red beets root
2 apples

Wash all ingredients and run them through the juicer. Run the pulp back through the juicer a second time. Serve and enjoy.

Colorful Green Juice

This juice combination is loaded with vitamins A and C, calcium, lycopene, iron and potassium that are essential cancer fighting agents. It also prevents night blindness; helps lower blood cholesterol levels and helps reduce inflammation.

3 cups spinach
3 cups romaine leaves
1 medium tomato
2 medium cucumber peeled
2 medium skinny carrots
2 medium radish
2 stalks celery

Add fresh ground black pepper to taste. Wash all ingredients and run them through the juicer.   Stir, serve and enjoy.

Blood Booster

This juice combination contains bioflavonoids; plant pigments that may help prevent or retard tumor growth. This is an excellent source of essential nutrients which help control blood cholesterol levels, promotes normal bowel function and also reduce the action of platelets, the blood cells that are instrumental in forming clots.

2 oranges
3 pears
2 yams
2 cups grapes
2 apples

Wash all ingredients and run them through the juicer. Run the pulp back through the juicer a second time. Serve and enjoy.

Fruity Delight

This juice combination is low in calorie and excellent source of vitamins B, C, beta carotene, folate, thiamine and potassium which help protect against cell damage by the free radicals produced when oxygen is burned in the human body, as well as help reduce the risk of certain cancers, heart attacks, and strokes.

¼ watermelon
1 lemon
6 oranges
2 cups pineapple
2 bananas
Wash all ingredients and run them through the juicer.   Stir, serve and enjoy.

Delightfully Sweet Juice

This sweet smelling juice will give a much needed vitamin and mineral boost without the heavy calories. A good source of thiamin, riboflavin, vitamin A, vitamin C and iron, incorporate this juice in your juice fasting recipe.

1pc cantaloupe chopped
3 pcs sweet potatoes peeled
pinch of cinnamon
2 tbsp. sucanat

Wash cantaloupe and potatoes; process together in the juicer. Add the sucanat and cinnamon. Stir and enjoy.

Olympic Flavor

Coconut meat contains lauric acid, which helps fight bacteria from intestinal parasites and wards off countless infections ranging from HIV to the common cold. Coconut water helps the kidney and bladder maintain proper functioning. Spinach and peach are rich in fiber and potassium, as well as beta-carotene, an anti-oxidant that converts to vitamin A which is essential for healthy heart and eyes. Spinach is also loaded with calcium, folic acid, vitamins K, lutein, and iron. Combine these three and you have a nutrition powerhouse.

1-½ cup coconut water
½ cup young coconut meat
2 medium peaches
3 cups fresh spinach

Wash all ingredients and run them through the juicer. Run the pulp back through the juicer a second time. Serve and enjoy.

Optimum Drink

This juice recipe is a low-calorie antioxidant packed drink, ideal for juice fasting. The antioxidant vitamins and minerals in this fruit and vegetable combination offer protection against breast, colon and prostate cancers and help reduce LDL or "bad cholesterol" levels in the blood.

3 apples
2 pcs fresh green Chinese cabbage
½ tbsp. cinnamon
 2 tbsp. honey

Wash all the ingredients. Run them through a juicer. Take the expelled pulp and run it back through the juicer a second time to extract all liquid. Stir juice and serve immediately for the greatest nutritional benefit.

Cocoberry Softee

Coconut has many bioactive compounds that are essential for better health. Especially the cytokinins found in coconut water help slow down the effect of ageing; eliminate cancer-causing substances and prevent the formation of blood clot. Try Juice fast now! It helps build all body tissues, keeps the skin soft and smooth and help lubricates the various organs and joints.

¼ cup young coconut meat
½ cup coconut juice
2 cups blackberries
2 kiwi fruits
½ cup pineapple chopped
¼ pears

Wash all ingredients and run them through the juicer. Run the pulp back through the juicer a second time. Serve and enjoy.

Coco Loco Delight

Coconut, banana and spinach all contain the electrolyte potassium that help maintain fluid balance; promote proper metabolism and muscle function and help maintain proper function of kidney and bladder. The coconut meat contains lauric acid which is beneficial in fighting off infections. This juice can provide an excellent amount of calcium, folic acid, vitamins K, lutein, and iron.

1 cup coconut water
1 cup young coconut meat
2large bananas
3 cups fresh spinach

Wash all the ingredients. Run them through a juicer. Take the expelled pulp and run it back through the juicer a second time to extract all liquid. Stir juice and serve immediately for the greatest nutritional benefit.

Tummy Cleaner

This juice blend is an abundant source of antioxidants beta carotene, vitamin C and E. It also contains bioflavonoids and insoluble fiber that protect against cancer and helps regular bowel movement.

3 cups kale leaves
1 large cucumber peeled
1 large green pepper
½ inch ginger
½ tbsp honey

Wash all ingredients and run them through the juicer.   Stir, serve and enjoy.

Rootfruity Drink

This juice blend is an excellent source of vitamin C which is necessary to make and maintain collagen, the connective tissue that holds body cells together. It also helps to build teeth and bones, strengthens the walls of capillaries and other blood vessels, as well as promotes healing of wounds and burns. This juice drink also helps the body neutralize carcinogens by protecting its ability to recognize and eliminate malignant cells.

4 carrots peeled
4apples
½ Chinese cabbage
2 turnip roots

Wash all ingredients thoroughly. Put all ingredients together in the juicer, stir and drink.

Vege Warrior

This juice combination is a great source of vitamin C, B6, potassium and other minerals that may protect against cancers and help reduce blood pressure. It also possesses curative power for headaches, gout, inflammatory arthritis, edema and other painful conditions.

2 lemons
2 radishes
1 bunch beet
3 sweet potatoes
3 stalks celery
1 onion

Wash all ingredients and run them through the juicer. Run the pulp back through the juicer a second time. Serve and enjoy.

Veggie Alert

This juice combination is a beneficial source of beta carotene, vitamin C, folate, protein, calcium, iron, potassium. High in fiber, drinking this juice can prevent constipation, night blindness, lower blood cholesterol levels and prevent certain kinds of cancer.

1 head cauliflower
1 head broccoli
7 medium carrots
3 stalks celery
¼ cup fresh dill weed

Wash all the ingredients. Run them through a juicer. Take the expelled pulp and run it back through the juicer a second time to extract all liquid. Makes 20 oz of juice. Stir and enjoy!

Creamy Coco

Coconuts contain lauric acid which has antimicrobial and antibacterial properties. It can help treat asthma, nausea, skin infections, ulcers and other infections. Limiting your diet to juices from fruits and vegetables is a nutritious way to give your digestive system a good rest.

2 cups young coconut meat
1 medium mango, peeled and pitted
½ medium papaya, peeled and pitted
2 tablespoon flax seed

1 maca root
1 head fresh lettuce

Combine all ingredients and run them through the juicer. Stir and serve.

Sweet Yummy

This juice combination is an excellent source of beta carotene, folate, vitamin C, B6 and potassium. Drinking this juice can help ease headaches and other painful conditions, speed up convalescence, lower elevated blood cholesterol, prevent heart attack and protect against cancer. Add this juice in your diet fasting.

2 artichokes
2 yams
2 beets with green tops
1 ½ onion
1lime
½ inch ginger

Wash all ingredients and run them through the juicer.   Stir, serve and enjoy.

Toxic Cleanser

This juice recipe helps protect your liver against damage from toxins. The combination of fruits provide vitamin C, potassium, folate, iron, calcium, bioflavonoids and other plant chemicals that protect against cancer, heart disease and help the body develop resistance against infectious agents. This juice is also rich in vitamin A which helps maintain healthy mucus membranes and prevent skin dryness.

3 apples
½ cup grapefruit
2 cup acai berries
½ lemon
a handful of beet

Juice them all through the juicer. Stir and serve!

Powerful Tonic Drink

This juice blend is an excellent source of vitamin C, beta carotene and flavonoid anti-oxidants. Onion is an effective heart tonic by hindering clot formation. Garlic is a powerful antibiotic and anti-cancer agent. Ginger helps improve the digestion of proteins, protects against the formation of ulcers and reduces intestinal parasites. It is also effective in treating nausea and motion sickness. Combined with astragalus herb, mushroom and broccoli, it can help promote a healthy immune system and prevent cancer.

1 onion diced
8 cloves garlic, minced
1 inch pc fresh ginger, peeled and finely chopped
2 pcs medium carrots
1 slice astragalus root
1 cup fresh mushrooms
1 cup broccoli flowerets

Wash all the ingredients. Run them through a juicer. Take the expelled pulp and run it back through the juicer a second time to extract all liquid. This recipe makes approximately 16 oz of juice. Stir the juice and serve immediately for the greatest nutritional benefit.

Wonder Juice

This juice combination is packed with essential vitamins such as vitamin A, B6, C and thiamine which helps control blood cholesterol levels and prevent some cancers. These nutrients are also essential for healthy hair, skin eyes, bones, and mucous membranes.

1 sweet potato
4 oranges
1 cup strawberry
2 carrots
2 apples

1 papaya

Wash all ingredients and run them through the juicer. Run the pulp back through the juicer a second time. Serve and enjoy.

Wipe Out Drink

This vegetable mix is a good source of antioxidant vitamins A, C, E and K, as well as potassium, manganese, zinc and flavonoids that help block cancer causing substances and bolster immunity. This is an excellent source of beta carotene, a nutrient that is essential for healthy hair, skin, eyes, bones and mucous membranes.

3 cups spinach
2 medium carrots
2 medium beet roots
1 large onion
2 stalks celery
1 cup parsley
2 medium tomatoes
½ lemon
1 tbsp honey

Wash all ingredients and run them through the juicer. Stir, serve and enjoy. This recipe makes 26 oz of juice.

Tasty Tangy Kale

This juice blend contains lycopene and endolse, compounds that can lessen the cancer-causing potential of estrogen and induce production of enzymes that protect against diseases. This juice is a rich source of vitamin A, C, potassium and beta carotene which are beneficial for the heart and help in lowering the cholesterol level.

7 large kale leaves
7 large romaine leaves
2 large stalks celery
4 large carrots
1 inch ginger
2 medium tomatoes

Wash all ingredients and run them through the juicer. Stir, serve and enjoy.

Orange and Avocado Juice

This juice blend is rich in antioxidant polyphenolic flavonoids and contains essential fatty acids which are good for the heart and help reduce bad cholesterol. In addition to this, drinking this juice supplies you with dietary fibers which are good for your digestion. Also contains a high amount of vitamin C which helps strengthen the immune system.

1avocado
1 melon
1 orange
4 stalks of fresh cilantro

Add the peeled avocado and cilantro into a blender. Secondly, add peeled melon and orange into the juice press. Mix this with the avocado. Add ice cubes, serve cold and enjoy.

Tropical Sweet Magic

This juice combination is high in fiber and an excellent source of beta carotene, vitamins C, E, potassium and iron. It contains pectin, a soluble fiber that is instrumental in lowering high blood cholesterol. This juice can help protect against some intestinal upsets, and prevent urinary tract infections. Try this sweet and tangy recipe in your juice fasting.

2 peaches
1 cup pineapple
2 mangoes
1 cup blueberries
1 tbsp honey
½ inch ginger

Wash all ingredients and run them through the juicer. Stir, serve and enjoy.

Prime Memory Booster

This drink has a slightly nutty flavor. It is an excellent source of choline, vitamin B and minerals that help increase neurotransmitter acetylcholine substance responsible for improving human memory.

6 large carrots
4 stalks celery, with leaves
½ head cabbage
½ lemon

Wash all the ingredients. Run them through a juicer. Take the expelled pulp and run it back through the juicer a second time to extract all liquid. Stir the juice and serve immediately for the greatest nutritional benefit.

Thirsty Mint

This juice is rich in electrolytes and water content that can beat tropical summer thirst. This juice combination is an excellent source of Vitamin A, C, folate, potassium and iron as well as pectin that help control blood cholesterol levels and essential for vision and immunity. Added mint taste helps relieve fatigue and stress.

¼ watermelon
2 pears
1 lemon
1 handful mint

Wash all ingredients and run them through the juicer. Stir, serve and enjoy.

Green Carroty Juice

This juice combination is rich in antioxidants compounds, minerals and vitamin A, B-complex, and vitamin C. Drinking this juice can help in lowering blood cholesterol level, weight reduction, red blood cell production, anti-aging, constipation relief, sperm production, clear vision, growth development and controlling heart rate.

2 stalks celery with leaves
4 cups spinach
1/3 melon
3 carrots
2 apples

Wash all the ingredients. Run them through a juicer. Take the expelled pulp and run it back through the juicer a second time to extract all liquid. Serve and drink.

Tropical Smoothie

This juice combination is a storehouse of vitamins C and E, beta carotene, folate, niacin, iron and potassium that help prevent cancer as well as treat liver and intestinal disorders. This juice is high in pectin, a soluble fiber that is important in controlling blood cholesterol.

2 orange
1 cup gooseberry
2 mangoes

Process all ingredients in a juicer until smooth. Drink up and enjoy!

CamuCamu Fruit Mix

This juice combination contains no saturated fats but rich in pectin, a dietary fiber that helps lower blood cholesterol levels, decrease the risk of coronary artery disease and heart attacks due to atherosclerosis. Camucamu berries are rich in vitamin C which is needed for the production of strong connective tissues as well as strengthening the immune system.

5 pcs camucamus
3 pcs oranges
1 cup strawberries
2 pcs red apples

Wash all the ingredients. Run them through a juicer. Take the expelled pulp and run it back through the juicer a second time to extract all liquid. This recipe makes approximately 16 oz. of juice. Stir juice and serve immediately for the greatest nutritional benefit.